Lumbar Spine Surgery

Indications, Techniques, Failures
and Alternatives

Lumbar Spine Surgery

Indications, Techniques, Failures and Alternatives

Edited by

Joseph C. Cauthen, M.D.

Staff Neurosurgeon
North Florida Regional Hospital and Alachua General Hospital
Gainesville, Florida

WILLIAMS & WILKINS
Baltimore/London

Made in the United States of America

Library of Congress Cataloging in Publication Data

Main entry under title:

Lumbar spine surgery.

   A revision of papers which were originally presented in the Lumbar Spine Surgery Seminar in Gainesville, Fla. in 1980.
   Includes index.
   Contents: Lumbar pain/Joseph C. Cauthen—Lumbar spondylosis and stenosis/W. H. Kirkaldy-Willis—High resolution computed tomography of the lumbar spine/by Kenneth B. Heithoff—[etc.]
   1. Intervertebral disk—Surgery—Congresses. 2. Vertebrae, Lumbar—Surgery—Congresses. 3. Backache—Surgery—Congresses. I. Cauthen, Joseph C. [DNLM: 1. Intervertebral disk—Congresses. 2. Lumbar verterbrae—Surgery—Congresses. 3. Spinal diseases—Congresses.
WE 750 L957 1980
RD771.I6L856 1983   617'.56   82-11195
ISBN 0-683-01500-1

Composed and printed at the
Waverly Press, Inc.
Mt. Royal and Guilford Aves.
Baltimore, MD 21202, U.S.A.

This volume is dedicated to
Frances, Fran, and Joseph, and to my parents.
Their love and support made it possible.

Foreword

This volume is a revised, updated, and edited record of the proceedings of a symposium presented to a live and participating audience. The subject matter was limited to the surgical management of disorders of the lumbar discs and joints other than fractures or fracture dislocations. Each of the faculty was asked to deal with limited special segments of this limited problem. Moreover, the reader is necessarily deprived of the benefits of interfaculty debate which followed each presentation and which was, no doubt, zestful.

Concern that these limitations might project the faculty in a more partisan role than their eminent records so thoroughly justify has led the editor to invite me to write a foreword.

The papers are well written; they are stimulating, provocative, and informative. They will serve as a valuable reference for experienced spine surgeons. Yet, I must add that I do not find myself in agreement with all that has been said.

My experience, for example, indicates that psychosocial problems play a very important role in patient selection. Spondylosis is often a coincidental finding in patients disabled with low back and leg pain due to systemic and, at times, reversible disorders.

Computerized tomography has added greatly to the diagnosis of changes in the spinal canal and in the root canals. It does not, however, determine when the changes are responsible for disabling symptoms.

Gowers, in 1888, observed that spondylosis would offer a fertile field for the surgeon. The valuable experiences described here indicate that cultivation of the field is still under way.

It is exciting to me to note that in the multidiscipline approach to the problem of the lame back, the era of the spinal surgeon appears to be at hand.

FRANK H. MAYFIELD, M.D., F.A.C.S.
Mayfield Neurological Institute
of Cincinnati
Cincinnati, Ohio

Preface

This text offers a collection of chapters dealing with current topics in the field of lumbar degenerative disc disease. An attempt has been made to present a sequence favoring continuity, but each author has been encouraged to present his efforts so that his chapter could stand alone. The chapters were originally presented in the Lumbar Spine Surgery Seminar in Gainesville, Florida, in 1980, and considerable revision has been required as the field advanced in the intervening months. Analysis of the reasons for surgical failures and alternatives to surgery are included for the reader's consideration. The collective goal of the contributors is to reduce the chance for error in patient selection, in diagnosis, and in surgical technique.

Acknowledgments

The concepts put forth in this text are the products of many years of careful study by the authors and by their teachers of anatomy, physiology, pathology, and surgery. These few words of recognition are a meager tribute to those pioneers who have shown the way to discoveries elucidated in these pages. The greater tribute will come from patients whose lives may be improved by these efforts.

Special thanks are extended to Sandra Sharon, Elizabeth Fannin, Carolyn Nutting, and Hazel Sessions for their parts in the preparation of the manuscript.

Alice Reid, Editor, and the staff of Williams & Wilkins have been invaluable in their support and encouragement.

The support of the Directors of the North Florida Regional Medical Foundation is gratefully acknowledged.

Contributors

CHARLES V. BURTON, M.D., F.A.C.S.
(Chapters 11 and 12)
Director, The Low Back Pain Clinic
Sister Kenny Institute
Minneapolis, Minnesota

JOSEPH C. CAUTHEN, M.D., F.A.C.S.
(Chapter 1)
Staff Neurosurgeon
North Florida Regional Hospital and
    Alachua General Hospital
Gainesville, Florida

**BERNARD E. FINNESON, M.D.,
F.A.C.S.**
(Chapter 4)
Chief, Department of Neurosurgery
Crozer-Chester Medical Center
Chester, Pennsylvania

KENNETH B. HEITHOFF, M.D.
(Chapter 3)
Department of Radiology
Abbott-Northwestern Hospital Corpora-
    tion
Minneapolis, Minnesota

**WILLIAM H. KIRKALDY-WILLIS,
M.D., F.R.C.S.**
(Chapter 2)
Professor of Orthopaedics
University Hospital
University of Saskatchewan
Saskatoon, Saskatchewan Canada

PAUL M. LIN, M.D., F.A.C.S.
(Chapter 7)
Clinical Associate Professor of Neurosur-
    gery
Temple University School of Medicine
Philadelphia, Pennsylvania

ARTHUR A. MAUCERI, M.D.
(Chapter 10)
Internist, Consultant in Infectious Dis-
    ease
North Florida Regional Hospital
Gainesville, Florida

**HUBERT L. ROSOMOFF, M.D.,
F.A.C.S.**
(Chapter 6)
Professor and Chairman
Department of Neurological Surgery
University of Miami School of Medicine
Miami, Florida

**J. CARL SUTTON, M.D., C.M.,
F.R.C.S. (C)**
(Chapter 9)
Orthopaedic Surgery
Montreal, Quebec, Canada

**ROBERT WARREN WILLIAMS, M.D.,
F.A.C.S.**
(Chapter 5)
Chief, Department of Neurosurgery
Sunrise Hospital
Las Vegas, Nevada

LEON L. WILTSE, M.D., F.A.C.S.
(Chapter 8)
Clinical Professor of Orthopedic Surgery
University of California Medical School
Irvine, California

Contents

1

Lumbar Pain—An Overview

INTRODUCTION

The impetus for writing this chapter and indeed, for encouraging the assembly of the material in this book has emerged from 20 years of dealing with patients with lumbar pain secondary to degenerative disc disease.

As a house officer in a neurosurgical training program, later a faculty member, and now as practitioner, I have been impressed with the simple fact that the majority of patients with lumbar pain radiating into the legs are suffering from pathologic changes involving the spinal nerves. Very few patients with low back pain, and almost none with accompanying leg pain, have a neurotic basis for their complaints, although many may be depressed as a consequence of their suffering. The incidence of patients seeking secondary gain is significant, but their symptoms are readily identified and the lack of supporting evidence for pathologic changes can be documented by the newer diagnostic methods described in this text.

THE DYNASTY OF THE DISC

There seem to be two firmly entrenched axioms ruling the operative approach to patients with lumbar pain radiating to the lower extremities: (1) always operate upon a patient with an extruded disc fragment if symptoms are considered related to the fragment, and (2) never operate upon a patient with a normal myelogram, even if symptoms appear to be localizing.

These axioms are in full consonance with the dogma of the Dynasty of the Disc recently articulated and denounced by MacNab.[1] This thinking holds that all, or nearly all, lumbar pain radiating to the legs is related to dislocation of the lumbar intervertebral disc against the lumbar nerves. Exceptions are made for congenital, infectious, or neoplastic etiologies, of course. The first axiom is widely known and fully reliable. The second axiom has been soundly disproven with evidence that subarticular nerve entrapment beneath enlarged facets often exists in the presence of a normal myelogram and is a common cause of lumbar pain radiating to the legs.[2]

The era of the Dynasty of the Disc has been drawing to a close, coincident with the widening recognition that lumbar nerve compression may be secondary to degenerative joint changes, not just disc hernia. Ehni's authoritative review[3] of the historical development of modern concepts of lumbar nerve compression is of great interest in this regard.

DIAGNOSTIC CONSIDERATIONS

We have entered an era in which the practitioner treating lumbar degenerative disc disease is compelled to consider numerous interrelated causes of lumbar pain and associated leg pain, including lumbar disc hernia, lumbar disc protrusion, extrusion, and sequestration, central canal stenosis, lateral bony entrapment, developmental, traumatic, pathologic, and degenerative spondylolisthesis, and lumbar instability.

Epstein's landmark contribution in 1960[4] and his more recent review supply definitions of great usefulness and clarity. We are reminded that nerve compression associated with disc hernia can be reliably predicted by a positive straight leg raising test, but this finding, and reflex and sensory deficits are less likely to be present in subarticular entrapment.[5] Central canal stenosis usually causes back and leg pain with enough variability so as to seem related to anxiety or to vascular insufficiency, but the cardinal features of neurogenic claudication are characteristic—paresthesia and hypesthesia after exertion, followed by weakness in the legs, relieved by rest or spine flexion. Lumbar instability can be predicted by the presence of pain on weight bearing or axial loading, relieved by unloading or bed rest, and by x-ray findings of traction spur, abnormal flexion-extension mobility, disc space narrowing, and facet subluxation.[6]

As indicated by the contributing authors in this text, high resolution computed tomography (CT) will often prove invaluable when the cause of symptoms is not clear, despite adequate myelography. An impression is emerging that further technological advances in CT scanning will eventually make myelography obsolete. If screening capabilities rivaling myelography are available, this will be quite desirable as an alternative. As this improved diagnostic state of the art is approached, few patients will be relegated to the category of "low back pain of unknown cause," and the erroneous concept that disc hernia is the only cause of back and leg pain will be discarded.

PRINCIPLES OF TREATMENT

Having proceeded to the point where an active search for the causes of pain is initiated, one should ultimately come to a conclusion that nerve compression is present or not and that the spine is stable or not. The patient with no objective evidence for nerve compression or instability will eventually recover from low back pain, aided by anti-inflammatory drugs, gentle exercises, and reassurance. Recurrences will occur and should be anticipated.

The natural history of an unstable spine suggests that fusion is not always necessary, as indicated by Kirkaldy-Willis in Chapter 2. Normal restabilization, in his view, occurs

reasonably often. This opinion is shared by Goldner[7] in his observations on the role of fusion in unstable spinal segments. Burton et al.[8] have also suggested that dorsolateral fusion may have less application in degenerative disc disease. When instability is present, and symptoms are unrelenting, several options for fusion are available, as indicated by Wiltse (Chapter 8) and Lin (Chapter 7).

Decision-making for patient selection is improved by consideration of pertinent physical and emotional findings, as outlined by Finneson in Chapter 4. It is axiomatic that proper selection will lead to improved surgical results and fewer numbers of failed back surgery patients.

In the difficult question of selection of the proper level for surgical exploration, Rothman[9] recommends utilization of the following priorities:

(1) metrizamide myelography;
(2) neurological deficits;
(3) pain distribution;
(4) straight leg raising test;
(5) x-ray findings;
(6) discogram.

Routine x-rays, while valuable in proving existence of congenital abnormalities, tumor, or infection, have not detracted from or supported the determination of the presence of lumbar disc hernia. Similarly, lumbar discography is considered too sensitive and the resultant findings too widespread through a normal population to be of value in this regard, according to Rothman.[9]

In those clinical situations where the cause of lumbar pain remains obscure despite adequate myelography, CT scanning may be helpful in determining the proper level for exploration. Further, many advocates of lumbar discography believe that films made following direct injection of contrast material into the disc yields invaluable information, as shown by Shapiro,[10] Collis,[11] and Cloward.[12] After specific criteria for selection of the patient and the operative level are applied, it is essential that the procedure be done with *technique appro-*

priate for handling nerve tissue. Basic requirements include a dry operative field and absence of iatrogenic nerve compression or contusion. While easy to describe, these goals are not easy to accomplish. The use of a fiber optic headlight and 2–2.5 power wide-field loupes is invaluable in this regard. The writer's preference is to use the operating microscope with 300-mm lens for that portion of the procedure where nerve dissection is required or when disc material is removed for nerve decompression.

As advocated by Williams in Chapter 5, the adequacy of the procedure can be better assessed if illumination is optimal, vessels are protected, and structures are magnified. On numerous occasions, the author has taken a final look with the operating microscope only to discover small retained fragments of disc, remnants of the ligamentum flavum, or facet edge which one would assume would have created problems.

RESULTS OF TREATMENT

In an attempt at evaluation of results of micro-operative technique in nerve decompression procedures, the author reviewed his own experience as to outcome in 175 consecutive patients undergoing operations for initial lumbar disc hernia with associated nerve compression. All of the patients were followed 1–5 years before a determination was made. Results are based on Finneson's patient self-evaluation criteria (Chapter 4) and statements made to the author in follow-up visits. All procedures were completed with careful attention being given to short incisions, thorough hemostasis, optimal illumination and magnification, and complete removal of disc fragments. When necessary, medial facet edges were resected to allow ease of access to the intervertebral space, or to discover and remove medially placed or central herniations. End-plate curettage was avoided, but vigorous attempts at removal of disc material from the posterolateral quadrant and the disc center were routinely carried out.

In this operative series, results were classified by the author as satisfactory or unsatisfactory using self-evaluation forms in 142 instances and statements made to the author in 33 additional cases in which questionnaires were not returned. Satisfactory results included patients who returned to occupations not requiring significant lumbar exertional stress and housewives who had reduced or modified activity levels but were functioning without medication on a recurrent basis.

Results rated as unsatisfactory included those who reported no particular benefit from surgery, those requiring non-narcotic analgesic medications and those who could not return to work on account of pain.

	Satisfactory	Unsatisfactory
Patients	161	14
Percent	92	8

Four patients, self-evaluated as unsatisfactory after the initial procedure, have undergone a second exploration with removal of additional persistent or recurrent fragments. After 1 year of follow-up these patients now rate themselves as having a satisfactory result. This change favorably affects the overall percentage of patients expressing satisfaction (94%). Longer follow-up no doubt will show a degradation of these figures as the progress of degenerative disc disease continues, but initial results compare favorably with those reported by Williams,[13] Wilson,[14] and Goald.[15] It is the author's opinion that improved patient selection and micro-operative technique have been responsible for improved results.

The technique of nerve decompression by medial facetectomy or facet undercutting deserves more emphasis as one considers additional causes for lumbar pain radiating to the legs. The now familiar subarticular nerve entrapment can be alleviated by careful removal of the medial one-third of the superior and inferior facets with a small osteotome, sonic-powered curette or angled Kerrison rongeur. Patency of the foramen and lateral nerve canal can be proved by inspection and passage of a right-angled probe beneath the superior facet and through the foramen, as advocated by Kirkaldy-Willis in Chapter 2 and Burton in Chapter 12. The exposed dura should be covered with an autologous fat graft to retard the ingrowth of fibroblasts and reduce the incidence of epidural adhesions, as described by Langenskiold and Kiviluoto,[10] Mayfield,[11] and as strongly advocated by Burton in Chapter 12 of this text.

The findings of Burton and Kirkaldy-Willis regarding the causes of failed back surgery syndrome are of great importance. The observation that 50–60% of a population of patients with failed back surgery syndrome had unrecognized, untreated lateral spinal stenosis deserves careful attention, and should prompt re-evaluation of patients with continuing difficulties related to degenerative disc disease.

CONCLUSION

Recent advancements in theory and practice have led to a realization that disc hernia is not the only cause of lumbar pain radiating to the legs and that stenosis of the central canal and lateral recesses is of equal etiologic importance. Accurate diagnosis requires high quality water-soluble contrast myelography. In those cases where this is not helpful, high-resolution CT may delineate subarticular nerve entrapment and nonapparent lateral disc hernias.

Improved results are dependent on careful patient selection, superior diagnostic methodology, and operative technique appropriate for handling nerve tissue.

References

1. MacNab, I.: Nerve Root Compression Syndromes, Presented at Hilton Head Island Neurosurgical Symposium, August, 1980.
2. MacNab, I.: Negative disc explorations. An analysis of nerve root involvement in sixty-eight patients. J. Bone Joint Surg. 43A:891–903, 1971.
3. Ehni, G.: Historical writings on spondylotic caudal radiculopathy and its effects on the nervous system. In Lumbar Spondylosis, edited by P. R. Weinstein, G. Ehni, C. B. Wilson, pp. 1–12, Chicago, IL, Year Book Medical Publishers, 1977.
4. Epstein, J. A.: Diagnosis and treatment of painful neurological disorders caused by spondylosis of the lumbar spine. J. Neurosurg. 17:991, 1960.
5. Epstein, J. A.: The role of spinal fusion, Question 2. Spine 6(3):281–283, May–June, 1981.
6. Frymoyer, J. W.: The role of spinal fusion, Question 3. Spine 6(3):289, May–June, 1981.
7. Goldner, J. L.: The role of spinal fusion, Question 6. Spine 6(3):293, May–June, 1981.
8. Burton, C. V., Heithoff, K. B., Kirkaldy-Willis, W., Ray, D. D.: Computed tomographic scanning in the lumbar spine, Part 2: Clinical considerations. Spine 4(4):379–390, July–Aug., 1979.
9. Rothman, R. H.: The role of spinal fusion, Question 1. Spine 6(3):279–281, May–June, 1981.
10. Shapiro, R., Galloway, S. J., Goodrich, I.: The evaluation of the patient with a negative or indeterminant myelogram. Radiographic Evaluation of The Spine, edited by J. D. Post, pp. 603–608, New York, Masson Publishing USA, Inc., 1980.
11. Collis, J. S., Jr.: Lumbar Discography, Springfield, Ill., C C Thomas, 1962.
12. Cloward, R. B., Buzaid, L. L.: Discography: technique indication and evaluation of the normal and abnormal intervertebral disc. Amer. J. Roentgen. 68:552, 1952.
13. Williams, R. W.: Microsurgical and standard removal of the protruded lumbar disc: a comparative study: comments. Neurosurgery 8(2):422, 1981.
14. Wilson, D. H., Kenning, J.: Microsurgical lumbar discectomy: preliminary report of 83 consecutive cases. Neurosurgery 4:137, 1979.
15. Goald, H. J.: Microlumbar discectomy: follow-up on 147 patients. Spine 3(2):183, 1978.
16. Langenskiold, A., Kiviluoto, O.: Prevention of epidural scar formation after operations on the lumbar spine by means of free fat transplants. Clin. Orthop. 115:92–95, 1976.
17. Mayfield, F. H.: Autologous fat transplants for the protection and repair of the spinal dura. Clin. Neurosurg. 27:Chapter 19, 349–361, 1979.
18. Burton, C. V.: The role of spinal fusion, Question 4. Spine 6(3):291, May–June, 1981.

2

Lumbar Spondylosis and Stenosis

In this chapter, the nature of the degenerative process is presented. Application of this knowledge to diagnosis and treatment follows.

PATHOLOGY

The L4–5 and L5-S1 levels are the most commonly affected areas. Later, the original lesion spreads to involve the whole of the lumbar spine. Farfan[1] has emphasized the importance of the concept of the "three-joint complex" of two posterior joints and disc at each level. Changes affecting one also affect the other and vice versa. The alignment of the posterior joints at the lowest two levels permits more rotation than at higher levels. Recurrent minor rotational strains of posterior joint capsule and annulus fibrosis are the most common causes of the development of degenerative changes in these structures and in the joints. Compressive injuries, often apparently minor in extent, can cause fractures of the cartilage plates of the disc. This is initially followed by slow degenerative changes in the disc and later, by posterior joint changes (Fig. 2.1).

The Posterior Joints

The sequence of change is similar to that seen in any synovial joint: synovitis, synovial tags in the joint, adhesions between the joint surfaces, capsular tears, degeneration of articular cartilage, the formation of osteophytes, and fractures of a lamina near the joint. This may produce a permanent rotational deformity. Increasing capsular laxity allows an increase of laxity of the joint and this is followed by an increase in abnormal movement of the joint (Figs. 2.2 and 2.3).[2]

The Intervertebral Disc

As a result of repeated minor trauma, tears are produced in the annulus. The earliest of these are circumferential. As these enlarge and coalesce, radial tears are formed. Later, an enlargement of the tears leads to internal disruption of the disc. The interior of the disc at this stage is completely disrupted by a large tear that extends from front to back and side to side. There is loss of disc height and the annulus bulges outwards around the whole circumference. From this point on, there is further disintegration of the disc with progressive increasing loss of disc height. The opposing vertebral bodies are approximated, the disc is filled by fibrous tissue, and the adjacent vertebral body bone becomes sclerotic. This final stage is called "resorption of the disc" (Figs. 2.4 and 2.5).[2, 3]

Combined Lesions

As stated previously, lesions of one component of the three-joint complex affect the others, and vice versa. Three stages can be recognized in the degenerative process.

Temporary Dysfunction. During this stage, rotational strains traumatize the components of the joint, often producing minor tears. Overlying muscle is in permanent contraction producing a decrease in joint movement. Healing takes place after each episode of trauma but the resultant scar is less strong than normal collagen. With each new incident, healing is less complete and degenerative changes more advanced. The patient enters Stage II.

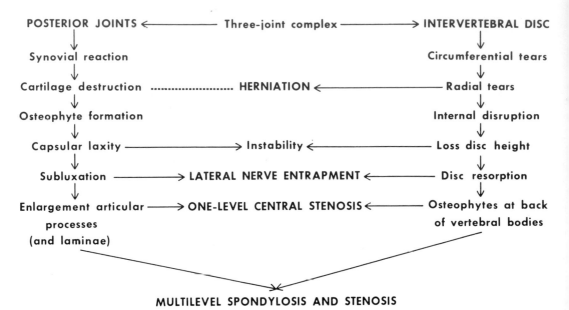

POSTERIOR JOINTS ⟵——————— Three-joint complex ——————⟶ INTERVERTEBRAL DISC

Synovial reaction   Circumferential tears

Cartilage destruction .... HERNIATION ⟵——————— Radial tears

Osteophyte formation   Internal disruption

Capsular laxity ———————⟶ Instability ⟵——————— Loss disc height

Subluxation ———⟶ LATERAL NERVE ENTRAPMENT ⟵——— Disc resorption

Enlargement articular ———⟶ ONE-LEVEL CENTRAL STENOSIS ⟵——— Osteophytes at back
processes   of vertebral bodies
(and laminae)

MULTILEVEL SPONDYLOSIS AND STENOSIS

Figure 2.1. The progression of degenerative change in posterior joints and disc with the interaction of the three joint complex.

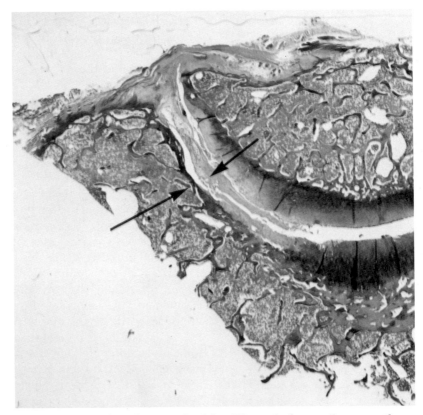

Figure 2.2. Histologic section of a posterior joint. The articular cartilage over the superior facet is eroded (*bottom arrow*). A large fibrous strand lies in the joint between the cartilage surfaces (*top arrow*).

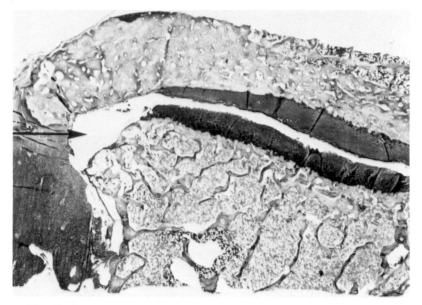

Figure 2.3. Histologic section of a posterior joint. The large clear space to the left of the articular surfaces (*arrow*) is due to capsular laxity—an unstable joint.

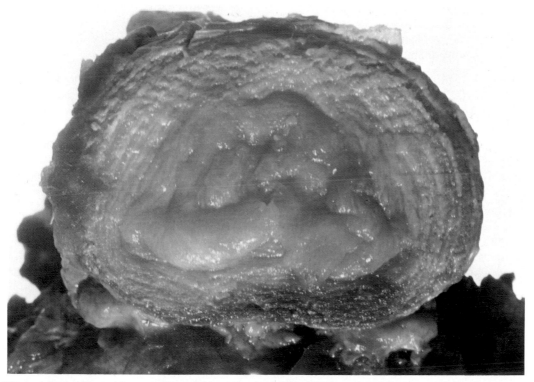

Figure 2.4. Transverse section of intervertebral disc. There are numerous small fissures in the annulus fibrosus. There is early disintegration of the nucleus pulposus.

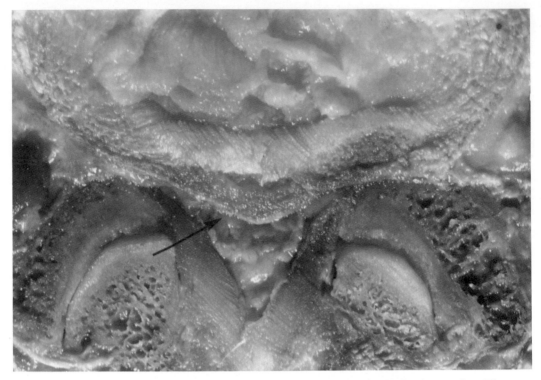

Figure 2.5. Transverse section of disc. The *arrow* points to a central disc herniation. There are several annular tears and disintegration of the nucleus pulposus. The central canal is small. The posterior joint cartilage is fibrillated.

Unstable Stage. Disintegration of the joint and loss of stiffness of the capsule and annulus permits progressive increase in the amount of abnormal movement. Anterioposterior radiograms, in right and left lateral bending, or lateral radiograms in flexion and in extension, demonstrate this increase of movement. A discogram reveals disruption of the disc. In the early phase of Stage II, healing can occur allowing the patient to return to Stage I (Dysfunction) but with further injury, the condition progresses again and healing is less complete. It is during the early phase of Stage II that disc herniation is most likely to occur. Later, with further loss of disc contents, the intradiscal pressure is reduced and herniation is less likely to occur. Finally, the patient enters Stage III.

Restabilization. Progressive disintegration of posterior joints and disc, loss of articular cartilage and of nucleus pulposus,

fibrosis around and within posterior joints and in the disc, and the formation of osteophytes produce a stiff joint. In this way, the abnormal movement of Stage II is abolished and the joint becomes stable once again. Recognition of these three stages is important in formulating a rational method of treatment.

One important result of this study of pathology is the appreciation of the fact that (1) a disc herniation seldom occurs without considerable previous injury to the annulus fibrosus and (2) that a disc herniation is often, if not always, accompanied by a lesser or greater degree of disintegration of posterior joints.

Lateral Lumbar Spinal Nerve Entrapment

Entrapment is a common sequela of degeneration of the three joint complex, usually found at the L4–5 or L5-S1 level. The sequence involves loss of disc height producing an increasing approximation of the vertebral bodies. This is followed by approximation of the bodies in the presence of posterior joint capsular laxity resulting in subluxation of the posterior facets. As a result, the superior facet moves upward and forward to narrow the intervertebral foramen and the lateral part of the nerve canal. The lumbar nerve that exits at this level is entrapped between the tip of the superior facet, the pedicle, and the back of the upper vertebral body. Occasionally, osteophytes project medially from the medial edge of the superior facet entrapping the nerve exiting one level lower.[2] Developmental anomalies may enhance this process (Figs. 2.6A and B and 2.7).[4]

Two types of lateral entrapment have been recognized. During the unstable stage, recurrent movement of the superior facet backward and forward may produce repeated entrapment of a lumbar nerve. This recurrent and dynamic entrapment may be produced by rotation or by extension of the lumbar spine. A second type occurs when the stage of restabilization is reached, and the deformity becomes fixed. Lateral entrapment is now permanent (Figs. 2.8A and B).[3, 5-7]

Central Spinal Stenosis

At first, canal stenosis involves only one level, most commonly L4–5. It is produced by the degenerative process referred to previously. In this instance, it is osteophytic enlargement of the inferior articular process that produces the stenosis. The inferior process enlarges medially to narrow the central spinal canal and to compress the cauda equina.[8, 9]

Multilevel stenosis usually follows. Degeneration at one level results in strains at adjacent levels. In this way, central and lateral stenosis originating at one level begin to involve other levels above and below the first level affected. Lateral stenosis and central stenosis can occur alone. In many cases of central stenosis, there is also lateral

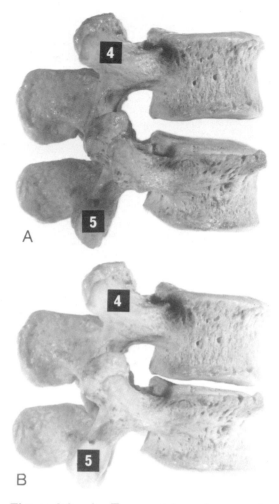

Figure 2.6. A. Two vertebrae in normal alignment. B. The same two vertebrae. Approximation of the bodies simulates disc resorption. The upper vertebra moves slightly backward on the lower and the foramen becomes smaller.

stenosis. It is not uncommon to encounter a disc herniation as a complication of stenosis.[8, 9]

Developmental Stenosis

When growth is complete, abnormal development of the different elements may lead to central or lateral canals that are more narrow than normal. Developmental stenosis alone seldom, if ever, produces symptoms. With an added small disc herniation or minor degree of degenerative ste-

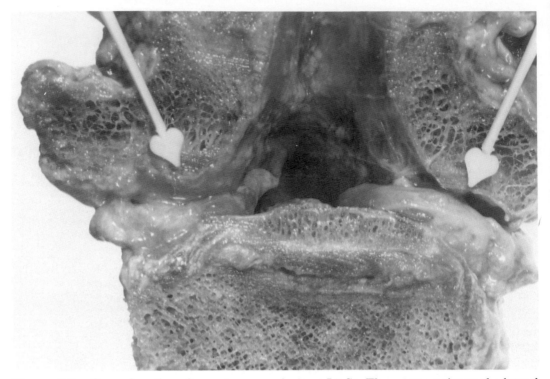

Figure 2.7. Coronal section of an autopsy specimen at L5-S1. The *arrows* point to the lateral canals. The canal on the left is narrow and the spinal nerve is entrapped.

nosis, symptoms may be produced. Thus, developmental stenosis may be regarded as an "enhancing factor."[4]

Direct Factors

Lesions such as trauma, spondylolisthesis, laminectomy, spinal fusion, Paget's disease, and fluorosis sometimes result in stenosis. Direct factors may be combined with developmental and degenerative changes in the production of stenosis.[10]

THE CLINICAL PICTURE

The symptoms and signs of herniation of the nucleus pulposus have been previously described by many authors. Central spinal stenosis is characterized by a bizarre picture. The patient complains of leg pain, made worse by walking and relieved by rest. The patient is able to work on a stationary bicycle, in the flexed position without pain, and may have night pain relieved by walking. Spinal movements are all somewhat diminished. Straight leg raising is diminished, but not as much as with a disc herniation. Sensory, motor, and reflex changes do not fit into the clear-cut picture presented by involvment of one nerve. Findings are variable, in both legs, with sensory changes involving one nerve, motor changes another, and sometimes reflex changes still another.

Lateral entrapment, without disc herniation or central stenosis, presents in a vague manner. Pain in the low back, buttock, trochanteric area, and posterior thigh is a common pattern. Sometimes, pain travels down the back or outer side of the leg to midcalf. More rarely, it goes as far as the ankle or toes. Spinal movements are painful and limited to a varying degree. Straight leg raising often is not markedly limited. Neurologic signs of involvement of one root may be present, but more often are not. The bowstring test is often positive, pre-

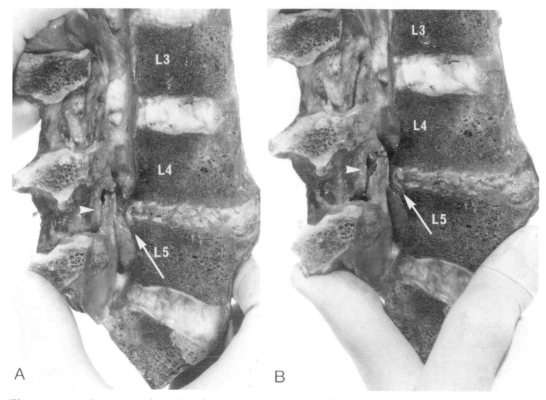

Figure 2.8. Parasagittal section of an autopsy specimen. The vertebrae are numbered. The *small arrow* points to the posterior joint. The *large arrow* points to the lateral canal in each picture. There is marked internal disruption of tbe disc. The posterior joint is markedly degenerated. A. Before rotation. The articular surfaces are closely opposed. The lateral canal is small. B. With rotation, the posterior joint surfaces separate. Tbe superior facet moves towards the annulus of the disc and the lateral canal becomes even smaller.

senting as tenderness on application of pressure over posterior tibial or lateral popliteal nerves at the knee joint level.

DIAGNOSIS

Plain radiograms are often helpful. Diminution of a disc space, the presence of vertebral body osteophytes, enlargement of posterior facets, and apparent diminution of the size of central and lateral canals lead to suspicion of disc herniation or stenosis. Marked diminution of the L5-S1 disc space with retrospondylolisthesis of L5 and sclerosis of adjacent vertebral bodies allows a high suspicion of lateral canal nerve entrapment.

Stress radiograms, with the patient standing, confirm the presence of increased abnormal movement, so-called "instability" (Fig. 2.9A and B).

A myelogram is often diagnostic in patients with a disc herniation or with central stenosis, but is only rarely of assistance in lateral stenosis. With the advent of the computed tomographic (CT) scanner, it is likely that myelography will be employed less often.

Electromyography and selective nerve blocks are of value in centers where there is a physician skilled in performing and interpreting these procedures.

The CT scanner, now of high resolution, makes it possible to diagnose a disc herniation and central and lateral stenosis without using an invasive technique. Assessment of

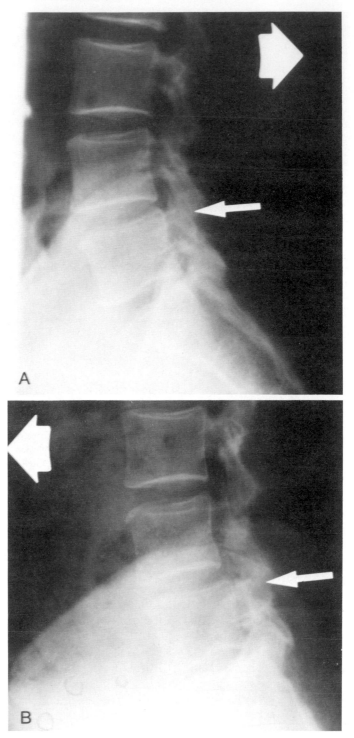

Figure 2.9. A. Lateral radiogram of lumbar spine in extension. Normal alignment of vertebral bodies. B. The same in flexion. Opposite the *small arrow*, the upper body has moved forward on the lower, a sign of increased abnormal movement—instability.

the mean density of an area enables the physician to predict with confidence that the image is due to disc herniation, cauda equina, spinal nerve, or scar tissue. In this way, it is now possible to diagnose the precise nature of the lesion in nearly every patient before any operation is done (Figs. 2.10–2.12).[5]

An increase in abnormal movement (instability), occurring usually at L4–5 and less frequently at L3–4 or L5-S1, is of great importance. As stated previously, it is nearly always possible to detect this by stress anterioposterior and lateral radiograms. Thus, it is necessary in diagnosis to assess two different aspects of the patient's problem:

(1) the precise nature of the lesion and

(2) the presence or absence of increased abnormal movement.

This is of great importance in making a rational decision for treatment, as will be seen later.

Differential Diagnosis

In patients with suspected central spinal stenosis, it is necessary to exclude (1) peripheral neuropathies secondary to diabetes, hypothyroidism, and alcoholism, (2) motor neurone disease, (3) vascular claudication, and (4) spinal tumors including secondary metastases. In cases of suspected lateral stenosis, the physician must exclude (1) posterior joint syndromes, (2) sacroiliac syndromes, 3) the piriformis syndrome, and (4) the quadratus lumborum syndrome. All of these latter conditions may produce referred thigh and leg pain which may be difficult to distinguish from a neuritic type of pain secondary to entrapment of a main spinal nerve. Quite often, the only way to exclude these lesions and differentiate them from lateral entrapment is by attempted treatment by manipulation, mobilization, posterior joint injections, and by a program of low back care and exercises. This is par-

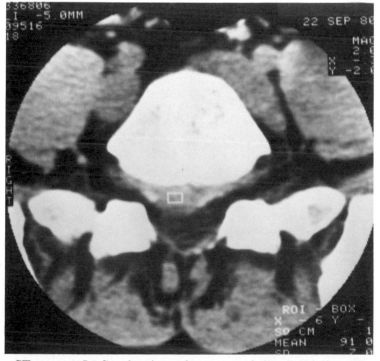

Figure 2.10. CT scan at L5-S1, showing a large central disc herniation. The censor (*white rectangle*) in the substance of the herniation indicates a mean density of 91.0 compatible with that of a herniation.

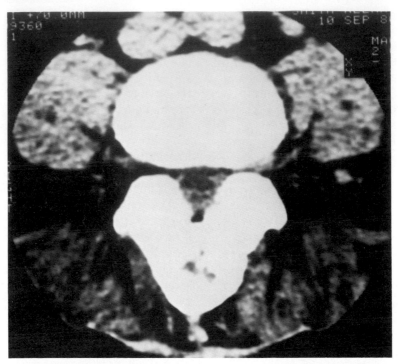

Figure 2.11. CT scan at L4–5. After a posterior fusion some years previously, there is marked stenosis of both the central and the lateral canals.

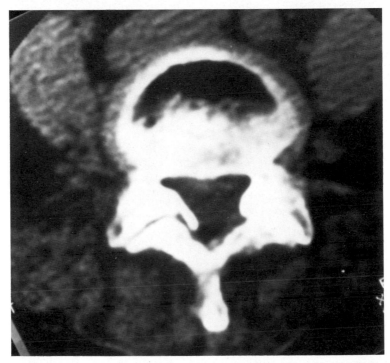

Figure 2.12. CT scan at L4–5. On the *left*, a large osteophyte protruded medially and backward from the superior facet. This reduces the size of the central canal.

ticularly difficult in patients with minor symptoms. In these patients, a cure often is achieved without making a precise and accurate diagnosis. This is satisfying for the patient and for those responsible for the public purse, but less so for the physician. A particular problem is presented by the fact that it is change in the posterior joint that produces lateral stenosis. Either the posterior joint, the lateral entrapment, or both of these may be the cause of the patient's leg pain.

CONSERVATIVE TREATMENT

In those patients with lesions of mild to moderate degree, in whom the pain, muscle weakness, and sensory changes are not severe, a nonoperative regimen is usually preferable.

Important aspects of this regimen include instruction in low back care, correct posture, an exercise program, and an exercise promotor.

Instruction in low back care is of great importance. Included is information about the structure of the lumbar spine, the type of lesion involved, the reasons why this causes pain, the activities of daily living, and rules for implementation.

Posture is most important. The symptoms and signs of spondylosis are usually aggravated by extension; thus, the patient should learn to assume a position of flexion for standing, walking, sitting, and lying. In achieving this, pelvic tilting exercises are of great assistance.

An exercise program to develop the abdominal muscles—the spinal flexor muscles—should be carried out on at least two occasions for 10 minutes each day. These movements are aided by the use of a light garment of two-way stretch elastic material (Camp Company Model 400). This exercise promoter gives useful support, aids flexion by pulling in the abdominal muscles, and does not allow muscle atrophy to occur because full movements of the lumbar spine are possible while wearing it.

Manipulation and mobilization help many patients with less severe symptoms and signs. These should only be performed by a skilled practitioner.

Posterior joint injections help many patients with a syndrome involving mainly the joints.

Chemonucleolysis is a controversial topic, but no discussion of the treatment of lumbar spondylosis is complete without reference to it. Injection of the enzyme, chymopapain, into the disc is intended to induce depolymerization of mucopolysaccharides and shrinkage of that part of the nucleus and annulus that is protruding as a herniation. It is unlikely to be beneficial when disc material is extruded and lying in the spinal canal. Injection of several discs has brought this modality into disrepute. The author considers it essential to perform a CT scan to exclude lateral stenosis before embarking on this procedure. When the patient's symptoms are caused by a simple disc herniation without central or lateral stenosis and in the absence of abnormal motion of the joint, chemonucleolysis seems a rational procedure.

Surgical Approaches

The thoughtful observer must be confused at the number of different procedures advocated and by the boundless enthusiasm exhibited by their proponents. One is, at times, almost driven to the opinion that the chief reason for embarking on a certain operation is that the surgeon has considerable experience in its performance. This comment applies equally to microdisc surgery, to many different techniques for dealing with a disc herniation, to decompressive procedures for the relief of symptoms in central and lateral stenosis, and to posterior, posterolateral, and anterior and posterior interbody fusions. It is, at the present time, more necessary than ever to attempt to formulate a logical approach in making the decision as to what type of operation should be done.

Before any operative intervention, it is essential to have a careful assessment by a well-trained psychologist. The assessment should include the Minnesota Multiphasic Personality Inventory and a personal interview. The psychologist and the surgeon should discuss the problem and decide together whether an operation should be performed or not.

Microsurgery on the disc cannot be condemned out of hand, but it cannot be recommended for every type of lesion in the central or lateral spinal canals. When treating an uncomplicated disc herniation, after an adequate period of conservative treatment, it is reasonable to have recourse to this procedure. The aim must be to remove a mass—the herniation—that is entrapping a spinal nerve and no more than this. To make certain that the lesion is not more than a disc herniation, it is essential to have a CT scan before embarking on this type of operation.

For any open operation, bleeding is reduced by positioning the patient on a frame that leaves the abdomen free from pressure. Hemorrhage within the spinal canal is controlled by avoiding injury to the extradural veins, by application of cotton pledgets, and by the use of bipolar cautery. Adequate lighting is obtained by the surgeon wearing a headlight. Visualization of blood vessels and nerves is made easier by the use of magnifying lenses attached to the surgeon's glasses. This first exploratory operation affords the greatest chance of success and, therefore, should be done with great care and attention to detail.

Discectomy

Many modifications in the technique of discectomy have been devised. Space does not permit more than a limited reference to certain important points. The exposure must be sufficient to permit the surgeon to see both the disc and the adjacent nerve and to retract the nerve with gentleness. After removal of the herniation, it is wise to pass a gauge* into the lateral canal to accurately assess its size. The gauge should be passed above or below, but not posterior to, the nerve in this maneuver. The gauges used are 2, 3, 4, and 5 mm in diameter. A canal of 5 mm is normal and one of 4 mm is borderline. One of 3 mm is definitely small. A narrow canal, not an infrequent complication of a herniation, should be widened to at least 6 mm in diameter. At the end of the procedure, a free fat graft from subcutaneous tissue should be placed posterior to the dura to prevent adhesions.

Decompression of Spinal Stenosis, Width of Laminectomy

A bilateral exposure is required. After removal of the spinous process, the ligamentum flavum is exposed and cleared of fat. The lower one-third of the upper lamina is removed after separating the ligamentum flavum from its undersurface. The central portion of the ligament on both sides is then removed. At this point, the lateral extensions of the ligament can be freed from the posterior articular processes by blunt dissection. The lateral recess both above and below the nerve that exits at the level concerned is then measured, as described previously. The medial one-third of the inferior articular process is removed using a small osteotome and mallet until the articular cartilage of the superior articular process is seen. This maneuver can be performed lateral to the ligamentum flavum or, after careful removal of its lateral extension, with scalpel and scissors. It is nearly always necessary, even when the stenosis is entirely central, to remove a portion from the medial aspect of the superior articular process. In dealing with lateral canal entrapment, it is necessary to remove the medial one-third of the superior articular process and to enlarge the lateral canal as far as the foramen, if there is any narrowing in this part of the canal. Removal

---

* Available from the author.

of the medial one-third of the superior articular process and enlargement of the nerve canal to the foramen can be done safely and easily with a Sonic Tool† using a curette or with Kerrison forceps. The nerve is identified and gently retracted and bone is removed, little by little, by rotating the curette and working away from the nerve, until the canal is 6 mm in diameter.

Length of Laminectomy

Laminectomy should be as short as is required to deal with the pathology, but long enough to remove all causes of cauda equina and nerve compression. If care is taken to remove no more than the medial one-third of the articular processes, a long laminectomy is not more likely to result in instability than a short one. Central and lateral stenosis, at one level, can be decompressed by a bilateral minimal partial laminotomy. In this, the central portion of the ligamentum flavum, the lower one-third of the lamina above and one-fourth of the lamina below are removed. This gives adequate exposure. To treat stenosis at two levels, a bilateral laminectomy at two levels may be required. Occasionally a three- and, rarely, a four-level laminectomy is indicated. Neither the decision to operate nor the length of the laminectomy should be made on the basis of the myelogram or scan alone. These findings must be correlated with the clinical findings. Whenever possible at the end of the decompression, there should be normal pulsation of the dura. If after a decompression at the L4 and L5 levels there is no pulsation, it is often considered wise to remove the lamina of L3 and even that of L2 until pulsation is demonstrated.

Avoidance of hematoma formation is very important. At this point, the wound is inspected for hemorrhage; it is controlled using bipolar cautery for intraspinal vessels, bone wax and cautery for extraspinal ves-

† Available from Quintron, Inc., 127 Holmes St., Galena, OH 43021.

sels. Free fat grafts 4–5 mm thick are obtained either from subcutaneous fat at the edges of the incision or through a separate incision over one iliac crest. These then are placed posterior to the dura to prevent adhesions of the paraspinal muscles to this structure. The wound is drained with two pliable drains attached to a compressible suction device.

The patient is allowed out of bed on the day after surgery. Thereafter, the amount of walking and other activity is gradually increased. He is able to go home between the 10th and 14th day. Before this, he receives instruction in care of the back, in gentle exercises to strengthen the abdominal muscles, and in posture and pelvic tilting. A light elastic exercise promoter is prescribed for continuous wear at all times when not in bed. During the 1st month at home, the patient is told to proceed slowly and carefully but to increase the tempo of activity and exercises day by day. If at the end of a day the patient has pain, he should go more slowly the next day. Gradual increase of activity without pain is the aim. Before leaving the hospital, the patient is told that he may have pain for time to time and that this is part of the process of recovery. The patient should be seen for follow-up at 1 month and at 3 months. It is usually 3 months before the patient is fit to return to work. At this time, a careful assessment is required as to whether the patient can return to his previous occupation or whether he should be assisted in obtaining lighter work. It is desirable thereafter to see the patient once a year to evaluate his progress and assess the value of the operative procedure (Figs. 2.13 and 2.14).

Spinal Fusion in the Treatment of Spondylosis and Stenosis

For many years, it was standard practice to undertake a one- or two-level fusion for patients with severe low back pain who did not respond to bed rest, bracing, or a plaster jacket. Brodsky[10] has reported on the high incidence of postfusion stenosis. Surgeons

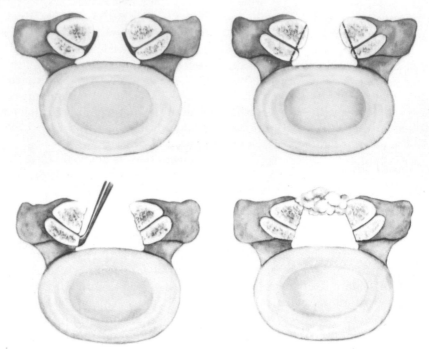

Figure 2.13. Diagrams to illustrate the steps of operation to decompress central and lateral canals. Laminectomy completed (*top left*). The line of section of the articular facets (*top right*). Removal of the medial and anterior portion of the superior facet (*bottom left*). The decompression completed: the lateral canals are enlarged. A free fat graft is placed posterior to the dura (*bottom right*).

I DYSFUNCTION	CONSERVATIVE

II UNSTABLE PHASE
  EARLY
 	
  LATE
	CONSERVATIVE
	
	FUSION
	DECOMPRESSION: FUSION

III RESTABILIZATION	DECOMPRESSION

Figure 2.14. Plan for treatment.

who treat low back pain are all too familiar with the patient who has had two disc operations, two or three attempts at fusion, and still has severe back and leg pain.

The proponents of posterior fusion, or posterolateral fusion, of anterior interbody fusion, and of posterior interbody fusion are not slow in their attempts to persuade us of the excellence of the particular operation that they advocate. It is, however, difficult to come to an impartial conclusion as to the efficacy of these procedures.

Undoubtedly, the role of the fusion in the treatment of back and leg pain is one of the most difficult problems confronting the neurosurgeon and the orthopaedic surgeon. An objective attempt must be made to identify the patient in whom a spinal fusion is indicated.

The decision hinges not on the predilection of the surgeon, but on the presence of increased abnormal motion in the posterior joints and disc at the affected level. The natural history of degenerative disease of the lumbar spine leads the patient through the early stage of Dysfunction to the intermediate Unstable phase to the final stage of Restabilization. It is in the Unstable phase that increased abnormal motion—Instability—is encountered. Lateral radiograms in flexion may demonstrate spondylolisthesis of one vertebra on the next (degenerative spondylolisthesis) and films in extension may show retrospondylolisthesis of one vertebra on the next lower. Most often, abnormal movement is shown by comparison of the flexion and extension films. Anterioposterior radiograms with lateral bending to left and to right may also demonstrate an increased abnormal movement. The term Instability has, in the past, been used to mean different things and, for this reason, the term Increased Abnormal Motion is preferred.

When this abnormal motion is present at the time of any operation to decompress the lumbar spine, it is wise to undertake a fusion at the same operation. This is usually a one-level procedure but occasionally it is necessary to fuse two levels. In some patients, there is abnormal motion without signs of nerve compression. Here, a fusion alone is all that is indicated. Figure 2.14

puts these conclusions in diagrammatic form.

The author prefers (1) to fuse the posterior joints and then (2) to do a posterolateral fusion. In fact, we do not yet know for certain which type of fusion is the best.

Failure of Operation for Back and Leg Pain

There are many causes—inadequate disc surgery, operating at the wrong level, recurrent disc herniation, arachnoiditis, and post-fusion stenosis among others. In our experience in Saskatoon, the two most important causes are (1) failure to diagnose lateral stenosis and (2) failure to recognize increased abnormal motion between two vertebrae.

References

1. Farfan, H. F.: *Mechanical Disorders of the Low Back.* Philadelphia, PA, Lee & Febiger, 1973.
2. Kirkaldy-Willis, W. H., Wedge, J. H., Yong-Hing, K., Reilly, J.: Pathology and pathogenesis of lumbar spondylosis and stenosis. *Spine 3:*4, 319, 1978.
3. Crock, H. V.: Isolated lumbar disc resorption as a cause of nerve root canal stenosis. *Clin. Orthop.* 115:109, 1976.
4. Verbiest, H.: Further experiences on the pathological influence of a developmental narrowness of the bony lumbar vertebral canal. *J. Bone Joint Surg. 37B:*576, 1955.
5. Burton, C. V., Heithoff, K. B., Kirkaldy-Willis, W. H., Ray, C. D.: Computed tomographic scanning and the lumbar spine II. *Spine 4:*4, 1979.
6. Schlesinger, P. T.: Low lumbar nerve root compression and adequate operative exposure. *J. Bone Joint Surg. 39A:*541, 1957.
7. Williams, P. C.: Lumbar spine, reduced lumbosacral joint space. Its relation to sciatic irritation. *J. A. M. A. 99:*1677, 1932.
8. Kirkaldy-Willis, W. H., Paine, K. W. E., Cauchoix, J., McIvor, G. W. D.: Lumbar spinal stenosis. *Clin. Orthop. 99:*30, 1974.
9. Kirkaldy-Willis, W. H., McIvor, G. W. D.: Spinal stenosis. *Clin. Orthop. 115:*2, 1976.
10. Brodsky, A. E.: Post laminectomy and post fusion stenosis of the lumbar spine. *Clin. Orthop.* 115:130, 1976.

3

High Resolution Computed Tomography of the Lumbar Spine: A Significant Advance in the Diagnosis of Lumbar Degenerative Disc Disease

High resolution computed tomography (HRCT) provides a specific, multilevel evaluation of bony and soft tissue pathology of the spine. It is a noninvasive outpatient procedure which can replace myelography and should significantly decrease the incidence of failed back surgery syndrome (FBSS). HRCT is capable of visualizing both the pathologic anatomy and the effect these lesions have on the nerve roots.

The findings reported here are based on over 3000 cases of HRCT of the spine performed by the author and his colleagues at Abbott-Northwestern Hospital and Sister Kenny Low Back Clinic Minneapolis, MN, in the past 18 months, and 2½ years prior experience with computed tomography (CT) scanning of the bony spinal canal. There has been excellent correlation between the surgical findings and the HRCT results. This procedure makes a significant contribution to the successful diagnosis and treatment of low back pain. Once the high resolution images are obtained, the success of the modality rests in the ability to interpret the scans and understand the configuration, appearance, and normal positions of the bony and soft tissue structures of the spine and their pathologic correlates. This chapter will review the technique employed, the normal anatomy of the soft tissue component of the spine, and the applications of HRCT in the diagnosis and treatment of degenerative disc disease, spondylosis, and stenosis.

TECHNIQUE

Adequate visualization of lumbar discs and other soft tissues of the spine requires a high resolution CT scanner with the capability of 0.8 mm resolution or less. Our patients are examined on the G.E. 8800 in the supine position. The knees are flexed to decrease lumbar lordosis. A lateral computed radiograph (Scoutview) is obtained for orientation and localization (Fig. 3.1 A). Using this image as a guide, contiguous 5-mm slices are obtained routinely from the midbody of S1 to the pedicle of L3 with no gantry angulation. The L3–4, 4–5, and L5-S1 disc spaces are covered (Fig. 3.1 B). No significant partial volume imaging problem is encountered with 5-mm thick contiguous scans.

In our experience, angulation of the gantry to attempt to parallel the disc space adds no additional information, does not make interpretation of disc pathology any easier, adds unnecessary time and complexity to the examination, and has the serious disadvantage of precluding image reformatting. Image reformatting is an integral part of our evaluation of the lumbar spine[1-6] (Fig. 3.1 C and D). Since contiguous scans are necessary for image reformatting, noncontiguous scans angled to be tangential to the disc spaces cannot be reformatted. In addition, noncontiguous examinations of the lumbar spine necessarily omit portions of the vertebral canal and a significant pathologic lesion or nerve root entrapment may be missed within the unscanned areas. Finally, images tangential to the L5-S1 disc cannot be obtained in most cases since the angle of the L5-S1 disc is ordinarily greater than the maximal 15° gantry tilt of the G.E. 8800 with imaging of the spine in flexion.

In order to detect bony stenosis and primary nerve root abnormalities of the S1 nerve root ganglia and S1 nerve roots below the level of the L5-S1 disc, the scan series is begun just below the anterior inferior aspect of the L5-S1 disc space to include the spinal canal to the level of S1-S2.

The routine technical factors for a lumbar spine HRCT imaging are: 400 MA, 9.6 seconds, 120 KV images using a scan field of 25 cm. The pixel size is 0.75 mm, and measured radiation dose is approximately 2.2 rads. Film images are obtained with a window width of 300 and a level of approximately 50 for soft tissue imaging, and a window width of 1000 with a level of approximately 134 for bone imaging. Initially, HRCT was performed following metrizamide myelography. Nine months of baseline comparison of the two modalities indicated that plain HRCT exams provided all of the necessary information. We believe that the risk versus patient benefit ratio so strongly favors CT that nearly all scans now are obtained without previous metrizamide enhancement, and myelography is used only in specific cases where HRCT and the clinical picture seem to disagree. Both hard copy film and TV monitor images are viewed routinely in the interpretation of the examination.

Full knowledge of the normal anatomic appearance of axial and reformatted images of the neural structures of the lumbar spine, and their relationships to the surrounding ligamentous and bony structures, is imperative in the interpretation of HRCT of the lumbar spine. While the normal anatomy of the bony lumbar spine has been well described in the literature,[6-15] the soft tissue component of the spine has not.[16-20] The advent of high resolution computerized tomography now allows the clear visualization of nerve roots and discs as well as other soft tissue structures (Fig. 3.2).

Within the interosseous segments of the lumbar spine, epidural fat fills the subarticular recesses (lateral recesses) and nerve root canals and surrounds the thecal sac and nerve roots (Fig. 3.2 C, D, I, and J). Axial HRCT images depict the normal subarticular recess as a triangular area adjacent to the thecal sac (Figs. 3.2 B, G, and H). The nerve roots course through this space and the inherent high contrast between the low attenuation fat (minus 100 Houndsfield units) and the neural elements, bony, ligamentous and soft tissue structures clearly depicts encroachment on this space and on the nerve roots by surrounding pathologic structures. This fat is the key to the high degree of sensitivity and specificity of HRCT in detecting entrapment of lumbar nerve roots by disc protrusion and pathologic overgrowth of adjacent bony and ligamentous structures. The boundaries of the subarticular gutter are formed posterolaterally by the superior articular processes (SAPs) and lamina, medially by the thecal sac, and anteriorly and anterolaterally by the vertebral body and disc (Fig. 3.2 B, C, G, and H). The superior extent of epidural fat at each interosseous vertebral level is the point of emergence of the nerve root from the thecal sac (Fig. 3.2 G and H). Within the intraosseous segment, there may be no epidural fat and the central spinal canal may be filled entirely by thecal sac (Figs. 2.3 H and I and 3.3 B and D).

At all levels of the lumbosacral spine, the nerve roots emerge from the anterolateral aspect of the thecal sac. Because they are surrounded by the low density fat, they are clearly imaged as they emerge from the thecal sac (Fig. 3.2 C, G, and L), course within the subarticular gutter (Fig. 3.2 E, F, G, K, and L), and exit the nerve root canal (Fig. 3.2 C–D and I–J). At the upper lumbar levels, L3–4 and L4–5, the nerve roots exit immediately under the pedicle. Axial HRCT images of the normal nerve root ganglia show them to be round in appearance and lying within the nerve root canal immediately inferior to the pedicle and the superior aspect of the intervertebral nerve root canal (Fig. 3.2 K). The postganglionic portion of the nerve root is oblong in appearance as it arises from the ganglion. It becomes linear as it emerges from the foramen and enters the retroperitoneal space to course inferiorly and laterally (Fig. 3.2 I and J). The nerve root ganglion itself, which is most vulnerable to impingement and ischemia, may be compressed by either lateral bony stenosis or a lateral herniated disc. Since the nerve root lies immediately inferior to the pedicle, some distance cephalad to the disc, the exiting nerve root and nerve root ganglia ordinarily are not compressed by a bulging disc at that level.

Care must be given in the interpretation of an apparent flattening of the lateral aspect of the nerve root ganglion, since it normally assumes an oval configuration as it merges with the nerve root. The close proximity of the ganglion to the pedicle above may result in partial volume imaging with inclusion of the ganglion and pedicle within the same scan thickness and, more inferiorly, the ganglion and nerve root.

Absolute measurements of the bony spine are relatively less important with HRCT than with other diagnostic modalities because of the ability to image directly the soft tissues of the spine and the relationship of the neural elements of the spinal canal to their surrounding structures. For example, absolute measurements may show a narrowed L3–4 nerve root canal through which a small L3 nerve root may course without pathologic sequela, while an abnormally large nerve root (i.e., a conjoint root) may be significantly compressed. The normal nerve root is surrounded by fat as it courses through the subarticular recess and nerve root canal (Fig. 3.3 A and C), whereas pathologic flattening of the nerve root ganglion or nerve root is associated with displacement or effacement of the epidural fat (Figs. 3.5 and 3.25). If the nerve root is surrounded by fat throughout its course in the nerve root canal, pathologic encroachment is not believed to be present (Fig. 3.6).

Asymmetry of the outlines of the nerve root and nerve root sheath complex may be due simply to a normal asymmetry of the nerve root sheaths (Fig. 3.4 A and B). When enlargement of the nerve is due to a pathologic process, the lesion should also be visualized.

The borders of the normal intervertebral nerve root canal are formed superiorly by the pedicle and inferior facet of the vertebra above, inferiorly and posteriorly by the pedicle and superior articular process of the vertebra below, and ventrally by the vertebral body and the intervertebral disc (Figs. 3.2 C, D, I, and J and 3.3 A and C).

The anatomic relationships of the L5-S1 level are dissimilar to higher spinal levels. The course of the L5 nerve root is oriented in a more cephalocaudad direction as it exits the inferior aspect of the L5 vertebral body and L5-S1 nerve root canal (Fig. 3.2 A–C). The inferior aspect of the L5 vertebral body widens considerably as it merges with the L5-S1 nerve root canal and becomes trefoil in approximately 14% of cases (Fig. 3.2 E and F). The exiting L5 nerve root therefore passes immediately adjacent to the L5-S1 disc as it emerges from the foramen of the L5-S1 nerve root canal. A disc, bulging laterally, may impinge on or displace the L5 nerve root. At spinal levels superior to the L5-S1 level, the ganglia and nerve roots exit the very superior aspect of the foramen while the disc lies at the caudal end of the foramen (Fig. 3.2 I and K). Therefore, simple bulging of the disc annulus does not entrap or impinge on the exiting nerve root at these higher levels. A pathologic bulging disc, however, may contribute to narrowing of the subarticular gutter and may cause impingement of the nerve root which is crossing that disc space to exit at the next lower level. This most often involves the S1 nerve root at the L5-S1 level[21-24] (Figs. 3.2 B, 3.6, and 3.17).

The S1 nerve roots course inferiorly within the vertebral canal of the S1 vertebra to emerge from the anterior sacral foramina at S1-S2. The S1 nerve root ganglion lies approximately 1–1.5 cm distal to the emergence of the S1 nerve root from the thecal sac, and medial to the S1 pedicle and base of the S1 superior articular facet. The central canal of the high S1 level is normally triangular in configuration. Medial overgrowth of the base of the superior articular facet, singly or in conjunction with protrusion of the L5-S1 disc may produce entrapment of the S1 nerve root in the subarticular gutter (Fig. 3.17). To ensure inclusion of this area within the scan series, the scan is begun 1.0 cm caudal to the anterosuperior aspect of the L5-S1 disc. Because of the angulation of the sacrum and the posterior location of the central spinal canal within the scan circumference, these axial scans pass through the central spinal canal at the S1-S2 level.

The anterior internal vertebral veins (AIVV) and radicular veins are key vessels in the evaluation of lumbar disc herniation. Both vessels are visualized on HRCT scan images. The AIVV are seen as small rounded structures in the anterolateral aspect of the central spinal canal in intimate association to the posterior aspect of the vertebral body and intervertebral discs. They lie anteromedial to the nerve roots in the subarticular gutter. These vessels may be large and measure up to one-third of the size of the emerging nerve root[25] (Fig. 3.6). These vessels connect with the radicular veins within the intervertebral nerve root canals. The inferior radicular vein lies in intimate association with the nerve root ganglion (Fig. 3.6). The AIVVs deviate me-

dially at the level of the pedicle and connect via anastomosing veins at the level of the midvertebral body (Figs. 3.2 A, E, F, and 3.3 B). At the L5-S1 level, these anastomosing vessels may be very prominent and numerous. Since they lie immediately adjacent to the posterior aspect of the disc, they may obscure the edge of the disc and may make exclusion of discal bulge difficult. This plexus of veins is most prominent centrally as the veins emerge from the nutrient foramen of the vertebral body.

Compression of the AIVV by herniated disc and entrapment syndromes of the lateral recesses are easily identified by HRCT. Loss of visualization of these normal structures at the level of impingement and, occasionally, enlargement of the veins caudal to an obstruction (i.e., central disc herniation) are usual findings.

LUMBAR DISCS, NERVE ROOTS, AND SOFT TISSUE PATHOLOGY

Careful evaluation of the lumbar nerve roots is the most important aspect of the HRCT examination of the lumbar spine. Compression or deformation of the nerve root by pathologic soft tissues or bony structures along its course can be detected by noting the direct effects these pathologic structures have on the nerve root, i.e., flattening, obliteration, swelling of the nerve root (Figs. 3.5, 3.7, 3.8, 3.12 A and B). Nerve roots may be entrapped in either the subarticular gutter (Fig. 3.11) or laterally in the nerve root canal (Figs. 3.8 and 3.10). Normal anatomic variance in the size of the nerve root sheaths of S1 do occur and must be differentiated from pathologic swelling or entrapment of the nerve root. This differentiation may be confirmed by metrizamide enhanced HRCT (Figs. 3.4 A and B). Swelling of the nerve root and venous engorgement distal to nerve root entrapment are the most common causes of enlargement. The resultant edema may also produce a less distinct profile of the nerve

(Figs. 3.12 A and B and 3.18 B). Extension of postoperative epidural fibrosis on to the nerve root sheath (Fig. 3.13), conjoint nerve roots, infection and tumors of the nerve root and nerve root sheath are other causes of pathologic nerve root enlargement (Fig. 3.14 A and B).

The attenuation values of lumbar disc material are higher than those of the thecal sac and the neural elements within the interosseous segments of the lumbar spine; the epidural fat allows delineation of the margins of these structures. Pathologic protrusion of a disc, therefore, easily can be identified and differentiated from the adjacent thecal sac and nerve root elements with a high degree of sensitivity and specificity. Because of the presence of the fat, there is no need for enhancement by water-soluble contrast material (Fig. 3.18 A and B).

Considerable attention has been focused on the herniated lumbar disc as a source of low back pain since the entity was first described by Mixter and Barr.[26, 27] HRCT provides a direct means of imaging both normal and pathologic discs.

The use of a narrow window width (300 or less) in the production of hard copy images and in imaging on the CT console is essential to highlight this difference in attenuation values (Fig. 3.15 A and B). Wide window widths (1000) are useful in studying bone. This setting, however, may mask completely the subtle differences in attenuation values which may exist between the discs on the one hand and nerve root elements, thecal sac, and postoperative epidural fibrosis on the other.

Transaxial scans obtained at L5-S1 with no gantry tilt normally show a thin symmetrical rim of disc posterior to the L5 vertebral body. This occurs because of the angle of the L5-S1 disc with respect to the x-ray beam (Figs. 3.2 C and 3.3 A). This is not usually seen at the L4–5 or L3–4 levels because these discs are nearly parallel to the x-ray beam. If degenerative changes occur, the disc loses volume as reflected by

decreasing height (Figs. 3.1 A and B and 3.7). As this change progresses, the annulus tends to bulge circumferentially.[28-30] The posterior surfaces of the bulging disc may retain a concave posterior border or bulge convexly into the central canal (Figs. 3.9 and 3.16). At the L3–4 and L4–5 levels, the nerve root exits inferior to the pedicle, well above the level of the disc, and isolated annular bulging of the disc ordinarily does not cause compression of the exiting nerve root. A bulging disc may, however, cause entrapment of the nerve root traversing its posterior aspect (S1 at L5-S1) by contributing to narrowing of the subarticular recess. In the latter case, the nerve root is compressed between the disc anteriorly and the base of the superior articular process or lamina posteriorly[21-23, 31] (Figs. 3.9, 3.11, and 3.17). Disc collapse may occur without annular bulging and show degenerative fissuring, calcification, and formation of marginal osteophytes (Figs. 3.8–3.10).

Asymmetry of disc protrusion is the hallmark of the herniated disc and separates it from a bulging disc with an intact annulus. A bulging disc with intact annulus characteristically bulges in a symmetrical fashion. The classical herniated disc protrudes into the subarticular recess, flattens the anterolateral aspect of the thecal sac and compresses the traversing nerve root at the level of herniation (S1 nerve at L5-S1), and may produce swelling of this nerve root distal to its compression (Fig. 3.18 A and B). Epidural fat, which normally occupies the lateral recess and outlines the thecal sac and nerve roots, is now replaced by the high density herniated disc (Figs. 3.18 A, 3.19 A, 3.21 A, and 3.22). If the herniation is large, the traversing nerve root may not be visualized on the section showing the disc protrusion because of its being completely effaced between the herniated disc and the lamina or superior articular process posterolaterally. Thus, the triad of the herniated disc can be considered to be: (1) asymmetrical protrusion of high density disc material, (2) replacement of the epidural fat in the subarticular recess, and (3) displacement or flattening of the nerve root by the disc and swelling of the affected nerve root distal to the level of entrapment (Figs. 3.18 A and B and 3.19 A and B).

In our experience, asymmetry has been a finding of much more importance than the absolute amount of disc protrusion in differentiating between a symmetrical bulging annulus of little or no pathologic significance and a herniated disc. Free fragment disc extrusions may be quite small with no more than 2–3 mm of disc protrusion. These lesions are significant if they produce a mass effect on adjacent neural structures (Fig. 3.22).

A significant, symptomatic herniated disc will directly affect either the nerve root or thecal sac by displacement, indentation, or compression. This direct nerve root involvement is clearly demonstrated by HRCT, and must be sought assessing the significance of a disc protrusion. Posterior displacement or stretching of the nerve root without compression by the lesion may result in significant symptomatology (Fig. 3.18 A and B).

Differentiation between central disc herniation and annular bulging may be difficult. Central disc herniations tend to be triangular in configuration with a central apex, while annular bulging is circumferential, rounded, and symmetrical. Symptomatic central disc herniations tend to be large. They may occupy the entire central canal with extensive compression of the thecal sac (Fig. 3.21 A–D). Central disc herniations may also have a more acutely angled fragment at the superior or inferior edge of the disc, representing a free fragment (Fig. 3.21 C).

Extension of the visualized disc protrusion cephalad or rostral to the disc level indicates migration of the extruded free fragment. These fragments may be contained behind the posterior longitudinal ligament (Fig. 3.22) or may be free in the epidural space. Sequestered disc fragments lie at some distance from the disc space.

They are often irregular in configuration (Fig. 3.23). Chronic calcified discs have high attenuation values and are easily imaged (Fig. 3.24).

Lateral disc herniation into the nerve root canal may cause severe symptomatology by lateral impingement of the nerve root and nerve root ganglia. Since this does not protrude into the central canal, no deformity of the thecal sac is seen. A pantopaque myelogram is normal in most cases. A water-soluble myelogram may be normal or it may show subtle nonfilling of the affected nerve root sheath and swelling of the entrapped nerve root exiting at that level. HRCT easily demonstrates the lesion as a large, high-density, soft tissue mass which fills the entire nerve root canal. This extruded free fragment does not extend into the central canal and epidural fat can be seen between the herniated disc fragment and the thecal sac in most cases. (Fig. 3.25).

In patients who have not undergone previous surgery, a protruding disc is outlined by epidural fat and a definitive diagnosis of a pathologic bulging or herniated disc can be made with a high degree of accuracy. In patients with previous surgery, however, extensive epidural fibrosis may be present and replace the epidural fat that normally silhouettes the disc margin. This makes imaging of the edge of the disc and exclusion of the recurrent disc herniation difficult (Figs. 3.26 A and B and 3.27). The diagnosis of recurrent disc herniation in the presence of epidural fibrosis can still be made by utilizing the relative difference in attenuation values between epidural fibrosis and disc material which ordinarily exists. The usual range for recurrent noncalcified herniated disc material is 90–120 H.U. that of epidural fibrosis is in the 50–70 H.U. range (with the G.E. 8800 scanner). However, in the individual case, one is interested in comparing the relative differences in attenuation values of the pathologic lesion in question with those of known fibrosis and disc density in the same patient. A very narrow window width is essential for visual detection of these subtle differences in density. In some cases, one cannot discriminate between these entities on the basis of the visual image and reliance must be placed on the attenuation values of the pathologic lesion. Therefore, the use of these attenuation values is essential if one hopes to differentiate accurately a recurrent disc herniation from overlying epidural fibrosis (Fig. 3.26 A and B). There is some overlap of attenuation values between discs and fibrosis, particularly with small linear sequestered fragments in which there is partial volume imaging resulting in low attenuation values of the free fragment. The numbers given are only guidelines and, in any given case, the suspected herniated disc material should be similar in attenuation values to density of the anterior aspect of the disc at that level, or another level in that patient.

In order to determine the accuracy of HRCT in the diagnosis of lumbar disc disease, a prospective study of 297 consecutive patients having nonenhanced CT lumbar scans was performed. Of these, 78 patients were diagnosed by HRCT as having significant pathologic disc protrusion or herniation (Table 3.1). Surgical confirmation was obtained in 44 of these patients. Surgical diagnosis was in agreement in 40: there were three false positives and one false negative. This led to an overall accuracy of 91%. Significantly, the three false positive diagnoses were obtained in postoperative patients. Upon surgical re-exploration, only postoperative epidural fibrosis was found; without evidence of recurrent herniated

disc. Therefore, in the previously nonoperated patients, there were no false positives and only a single false negative (on review, the false negative was due to interpretive error and could have been avoided with utilization of narrow window widths). Of the three false positives, one is believed to have been due to misinterpretation of computer artifact superimposed on postoperative fibrosis which produced a triangular area of increased density in the subarticular recess. Additionally, this study was performed before utilization of the electronic cursor for accurate discrimination of the attenuation values of disc and postoperative fibrosis. Use of the cursor would have prevented the false positive diagnosis in two of these cases since the attenuation values of the questioned lesions were lower than that of disc material.

Since that study, attenuation values have been utilized to evaluate patients with postoperative epidural fibrosis and questionable recurrent disc herniation. An additional six patients have been evaluated in whom surgically confirmed recurrent disc herniation underlying the epidural fibrosis was diagnosed by HRCT. Significantly, the surgeon commented that the herniated disc was difficult to find in two of these patients because of very dense postoperative fibrosis which resulted in a difficult surgical approach and the procedure might have been terminated before finding the fragment if HRCT had not definitively localized the lesion.

The characteristic appearance of disc herniation on postmetrizamide scans includes protrusion of the high density disc, flattening of the anterolateral aspect of the thecal sac, and nonfilling of the nerve root sheath by metrizamide, on the affected side. Reformatted images may be helpful in delineating these abnormalities (Fig. 3.28). The excellent delineation of abnormalities of discs on plain, nonmetrizamide-enhanced scans, however, obviates the necessity for lumbar myelography and metrizamide-enhanced HRCT in most patients with lum-

Table 3.1. CT diagnosis of Herniated Discs: February–May, 1980 (78 Patients)

Surgical Confirmation	Patients	%
Surgical—HRCT agreement	40	91
False positive	3[a]	7
False negative	1[b]	2

[a] All false positive exams occurred in previously operated patients with postoperative epidural fibrosis.
[b] Soft disc missed because of wide window width setting.

bar spine disease. In our practice, myelography followed by enhanced HRCT scanning is only occasionally performed.

In some cases, epidural fibrosis is associated with arachnoiditis.[32] This is still best studied by means of water-soluble myelography. The changes seen in postmetrizamide enhanced HRCT scans include thickening, clumping, and irregularity of the nerve roots within the thecal sac. These nerve roots eventually become adherent to the periphery of the thecal sac (Fig. 3.29). Increased soft tissue thickness about droplets of pantopaque has been noted in several cases following meylography. These findings would suggest a local inflammatory response to the droplets of pantopaque.[33, 34] The nerve root sheaths of the L5 and S1 nerve roots area are the most common location for retained droplets of pantopaque following myelography. Surgically documented arachnoiditis within nerve root sheaths containing pantopaque has recently been reported. This lends strong support to the hypothesis of pantopaque-induced arachnoiditis.[35] Imaging of soft tissue (nerve root) thickening about the droplets of pantopaque within the thecal sac seems to be an in vivo confirmation of these surgical findings. On nonenhanced scans, one may see only a deformity of the thecal sac (Fig. 3.30).

Disc space infection may produce retroperitoneal mass effect adjacent to the disc space. This inflammatory mass may extend into the nerve root canal and cause enlargement of the nerve roots within the lateral recess of the central canal (Figs. 3.14 A and B and 3.31). Irregular erosion and destruction of the vertebral end plates is also seen.

Lumbar Stenosis

The pathogenesis of lumbar spondylosis and stenosis is believed to be due to recurrent rotational strains which result in simultaneous disc resorption, loss of disc height, and enlargement of facets.[36–45] Repeated rotational strains and other acquired insults and injuries, combined with normal aging, produce accelerated degenerative disc disease and degenerative changes in the posterior zygoapophyseal joints.[12, 41, 42, 46, 47] Degenerative changes in the disc inevitably cause degenerative changes in the posterior zygoapophyseal joints and vice versa.[41, 48] This concept of the three joint complex, proposed by Farfan, is well supported by experimental evidence.[37–40] It is essential to consider changes in the posterior joints and discs conjointly.

The causes of disc height loss are internal disruption, resorption, chemonucleolysis, and the sequelae of discectomy.[41, 44] The posterior zygoapophyseal joint sequelae which accompany disc degeneration and loss of disc volume are ligamentous laxity of the capsule, ligamentous instability, and posterior joint strain with subsequent overriding and subluxation of the posterior joints.[46] Later changes in the superior and inferior articular processes include hypertrophy and osteophyte formation reflecting subperiosteal bone deposition (Figs. 3.8–3.11, and 3.32 A-C). Enlargement of the inferior articular facets by these pathologic processes may result in central stenosis (Figs. 3.9, 3.35, and 3.37). Stenosis may occur either within the nerve root canal itself (Figs. 3.34–3.37) or within the subarticular recess (Figs. 3.9, 3.11, and 3.17). Degenerative changes of the zygoapophyseal joints accompany the previously discussed disc findings.[37, 38,41–45, 49, 50] The zygoapophyseal joints may be widened or narrowed and the joint surface may be irregular or frayed. Hypertrophic overgrowth of the superior and inferior articular facets, as well as osteophytes, are common evidence of the degenerative changes. Widening of the medial aspect of the zygoapophyseal joints may produce a "clamshell" appearance to the zygoapophyseal joint with the ligamentum flavum traversing the gaping medial aspect of the facet joints (Fig. 3.32 C). Asymmetrical orientation of the zygoapophyseal joints (tropism) and asymmetrical fusion are believed to be predisposing factors in degenerative spondylosis because of the production of instability and unequal stress loading[40] (Fig. 3.33 A and B). Asymmetrical fusion of the transitional vertebra, such as partial lumbarization of the first sacral segment, may also contribute to unequal stress loading and an increased incidence of low back pain. Bony entrapment of lumbar nerve roots involves three separate processes, occurring singly or in combination: (1) degenerative changes, (2) developmental changes, and (3) lesions that produce direct entrapment of the spinal nerves.[41, 51-53] Central and lateral spinal stenosis are not separate entities but rather are sequelae of the spectrum of spondylosis that occur at some time during the course of the above three pathogenic processes. Developmental stenosis may be asymptomatic until the secondary development of degenerative spondylosis or disc protrusion causes critical narrowing of the central canal (Fig. 3.39). Spondylosis and stenosis are not synonymous, however, and, degenerative changes may produce enlargement of the posterior articular processes without narrowing the central spinal canal or lateral nerve root canals.

Fixed lateral spinal stenosis with nerve root entrapment, either within the subarticular gutter or within the intervertebral nerve root canal, is more common than central stenosis.[48] Enlargement of the superior articular facet in conjunction with loss of disc height is a relatively common etiologic agent. As the disc loses volume, there is concomitant ligamentous laxity resulting in anterior and superior subluxation of the superior articular process of the vertebra below. As the disc space narrowing becomes marked, the superior articular process underrides the pedicle above, and entrapment of the nerve root exiting at that level occurs (Figs. 3.7, 3.8, and 3.10). Medial enlargement of the superior articular process may cause entrapment of the nerve root which has just emerged from the anterolateral aspect of the thecal sac and will exit at the level below, S1 at L5–S1[22, 23, 54] (Figs. 3.9 and 3.11).

In addition to pathologic enlargement of the superior articular processes, there is often associated degenerative disc protrusion and/or formation of posterolateral osteophytes which further compromises the nerve root canal and narrows the subarticular recess. The posterolateral osteophytes cause the normally rounded posterolateral margin of the vertebral body to have a more squared-off appearance. The osteophytes cause elongation of the nerve root canal and, in conjunction with enlargement of the superior articular process, may contribute to the stenotic process. When associated bulging of the disc occurs, it causes a sharply angled narrowing of the subarticular recess with entrapment of the nerve root (superior articular process syndrome) (Fig. 3.17). Focal osteophytes or herniation of a calcified disc may cause severe narrowing of the intervertebral nerve root canal (Figs. 3.8 and 3.10). More generalized spondylosis may involve the inferior articular facets as well and the production of narrowing of the central canal. In severe cases of generalized spondylosis, both central and lateral spinal stenosis may coexist (Fig. 3.37).

Lateral stenosis may be either fixed or dynamic.[41] Dynamic stenosis is thought to occur in those patients with ligamentous laxity in which rotatory motion of the spine causes anterior and superior subluxation of the superior articular facet. This produces impingement of the nerve root, either in the subarticular recess or intervertebral nerve root canal. To demonstrate this lesion, extension-rotation views of the lumbar spine are obtained following a routine study in flexion. This is performed by positioning the patient with the shoulders flat on the table and elevation of the ipsilateral hip. This reproduces the patient's pain, demonstrates ligamentous laxity with widening of the zygoapophyseal joints, and dynamic narrowing of the lateral nerve root canal on the side elevated. Impingement of the nerve root ganglion is evidenced as flattening of the posterior aspect of the ganglion by the superior articular process (Fig. 3.38).

Developmental central stenosis is recognized when the measurements of the spinal canal are smaller than normal at maturity. This more commonly affects the sagittal dimension of the central canal rather than the coronal or interpedicular measurements. The entire lumbar canal often is abnormal but a segmental narrowing may exist. At the time a symptomatic back patient is studied, it is difficult to determine whether this stenosing lesion was developmental or degenerative in nature because of the superimposed degenerative changes (Fig. 3.39). Where there is asymmetry of the lamina and facet joints, it is likely that the lesion began as a developmental abnormality. Symptomatic cases of developmental stenosis almost always are associated with secondary degenerative changes, with symptoms being attributed to further compromise of the central canal.

Degenerative central stenosis is evidenced either by disc protrusion, hypertrophic enlargement of the inferior articular facets and thickening of the ligamentum flavum with dorsolateral encroachment on the central canal, or projection of an osteophyte arising from the inferior articular facet into the central canal[31, 55-57] (Fig. 3.10). Patients with symptoms of central spinal stenosis often exhibit all three findings of bony hypertrophy, ligamentous thickening, and disc protrusion. The central canal in these patients is markedly diminished in size and is usually triangular in shape with outwardly concave borders (Figs. 3.9 and 3.40). The ability to image soft tissues better defines the pathologic narrowing which is present. The bony measurements may be normal in the face of severe central stenosis due to marked ligamentous thickening and disc protrusion.

Spondylolytic spondylolisthesis may produce direct entrapment of spinal nerves.[58] The hallmark of spondylolytic spondylolisthesis is the break in the pars interarticularis. The lateral computed radiograph demonstrates the break in the pars as well as the anterior and inferior displacement of the vertebral body above on the disc and body below (Fig. 3.41 A). This lesion most commonly occurs at L5-S1. There is usually bony and cartilaginous overgrowth involving the pars superior. As the vertebral body and the rostral portion of the pars interarticularis slip anteriorly and inferiorly, this overgrown portion of the pars comes to rest within the lateral recess with entrapment of the exiting nerve root, i.e. the L5 nerve at L5-S1 (Fig. 3.41 B). The nerve root is compressed between the superior pars and pedicle of the cephalad vertebrae (L5), and the rostral vertebral body and disc. At the level of the slip, the central canal and nerve root canals are typically elongate in the anteroposterior dimension. Hypertrophic changes of the inferior articular facets may cause narrowing of the coronal dimension of the central canal. Because of the distorted anatomy of the transaxial views, normal borders of the nerve root canal cannot be always identified. Sagittal image reformatting is very valuable in these cases for defining the anatomic structures and impingement on the nerve canal by the rostral portion of the pars.[5] The fibrous build-up of the annulus also is well visualized in the sagittal plane. Sagittal reconstruction through the nerve root canals can trace the course of the nerve root and conclusively demonstrate marked constriction of the superior-inferior dimension of the nerve root canal and definite nerve root impingement when axial images are indeterminate (Fig. 3.41 C).

Degenerative spondylolisthesis results in anterior slippage of the cephalad vertebral body on the caudal vertebra without spondylolysis. This entity most commonly occurs at L4-5. The lateral computed radiograph best shows the degree of anterior displacement. The disc space is often narrowed and axial. HRCT images demonstrate marked erosive irregularity of the zygoapophyseal joints with cupping, erosion, and enlargement of the superior articular processes (Figs. 3.10 and 3.12 A). Marked erosion of the anterior aspect of the superior articular process causes loss of support and allows the inferior articular process and vertebral body to slide forward *en masse.* No spondylolytic break in the pars interarticularis is seen. Because of the anterior slip of the vertebral body, the disc is imaged as an apparent broad protrusion in to the central spinal canal (Fig. 3.42 C). These cases exhibit severe productive overgrowth and fragmentation of the articular processes. The prominence of the disc, plus the severe spondylosis may result in the production of severe subarticular stenosis as well as central stenosis. Bony lateral stenosis is rare, however, degenerative fibrocartilaginous build-up at the margin of the disc often incorporates the exiting nerve roots, with loss of nerve root identity on HRCT images.[39, 59, 60] (Figs. 3.10 and 3.42 C and D).

Retrospondylolisthesis is demonstrated on the computed radiograph as posterior slippage of the vertebral body above on the vertebra below. The pathologic anatomy of retrospondylolisthesis is dissimilar to that of degenerative spondylolisthesis. The former is due to marked overgrowth and fragmentation of the zygoapophyseal joints and is associated with central and subarticular stenosis, while the latter most often is associated with lateral stenosis (Fig. 3.43). Posterior displacement of the rostral vertebral body causes the superior articular process of the caudal vertebral body to project both anteriorly and superiorly, impinging on the nerve root within the lateral nerve root canal (Fig. 3.43 C).

Computed tomography is an excellent modality for the evaluation of burst fractures of the lumbar vertebrae as well as suspected fractures of the posterior elements.[61] Disruption of the central canal and displacement of fragments into the central canal with compression of the cauda equina and lumbar nerve roots can easily be identified. An associated retroperitoneal or intra-abdominal hemorrhage can be evaluated simultaneously (Fig. 3.44).

The incidence of laminectomies in this country is 75 per 100,000, or approximately 155,000 laminectomies per year.[62] The survey of the literature indicates that the over-

all failure rate for low back surgery is approximately 25%.[63] There is, therefore, a large patient population who are either unimproved after surgery or who have recurrent symptomatology. CT of the spine offers a noninvasive, easily obtained method of evaluating bony and soft tissue elements of the spine for complications of surgery or residual or recurrent lesions.[64-67] More than one-half of our patients with FBSS have been found to have residual lateral spinal stenosis[7] (Fig. 3.45). Other causative lesions are postoperative epidural fibrosis (Figs. 3.13, 3.27, and 3.29), fibrosis plus recurrent herniated disc (Fig. 3.26 A and B), or recurrent disc without fibrosis (Figs. 3.15, 3.45, and 3.46) and fusion overgrowth (Fig. 3.49).

Placement of large volume free fat grafts at surgery dramatically reduces or precludes the development of postoperative epidural fibrosis. Postoperative scans up to 2 years following placement of the grafts show the grafts to be viable and essentially to retain their volume. There is an approximate one-third decrease in the size of the graft over time and, therefore, large fat grafts are placed (Fig. 3.47). In some cases, a pseudomembrane forms posterior to the fat graft which simulates ligamentum flavum[46, 68] (Fig. 3.48).

Fusion overgrowth may produce central or lateral spinal stenosis[47, 69] (Fig. 3.49). In postoperative scans, patients with spinal fusion also may demonstrate either fusion failure or solid fusion bone which bridges the area of instability (Fig. 3.50). Finally, HRCT can provide an immediate postoperative evaluation of the completeness of disc resection and relief of soft tissue and bony entrapment (Fig. 3.51 A–C). The improved understanding of the anatomy of the spine and lesions affecting it afforded by HRCT can be used to evaluate new surgical techniques devised to relieve the pathology without producing instability.[66, 67, 70, 71] In light of the stated advantages of HRCT, it is evident that HRCT of the spine will lead to a greatly decreased incidence of failed back surgery syndrome in the future, by providing a more complete understanding of the entire pathologic process prior to the first surgical procedure.

SUMMARY

High resolution computed tomography of the lumbar spine has led to a dramatic expansion of the understanding and knowledge of the normal and pathologic anatomy of the lumbar spine. The author considers HRCT to be the diagnostic radiologic procedure of choice in the evaluation of patients with low back pain and sciatica. With the use of HRCT, water-soluble contrast myelography can be relegated to a secondary procedure being performed only in complex and diagnostically difficult cases when plain CT and the clinical picture seem to disagree. The most common cause of failed back surgery syndrome has been the lack of adequate information prior to the first surgical procedure.[72] HRCT provides an accurate means of preoperatively assessing both the bony and soft tissue pathology of the spine. HRCT is capable of directly visualizing not only the pathologic processes affecting the spine but also the direct effect these lesions may have on the nerve roots and thecal sac. HRCT provides direct evidence of nerve root involvement by bony stenosis, herniated disc, and postoperative perineural fibrosis. HRCT provides very clear images of the bony spinal and intervertebral nerve root canals, as well as the soft tissue occupying those spaces, identifies herniated and sequestered discs, differentiates the various causes of failed back surgery syndrome (recurrent disc, fibrosis, stenosis, fusion overgrowth, etc.), and defines nerve root entrapment more accurately than any other current imaging modality used in the study of lumbar spine disease.

Thus, use of current HRCT technology with its increased capability for accurate interpretation and diagnosis, can be reasonably expected to reduce significantly the incidence of the failed back surgery syndrome. Coronal, sagittal, off-axis reformatted images, and other software advances promise even more sophisticated and accurate evaluation of the spine in the future.

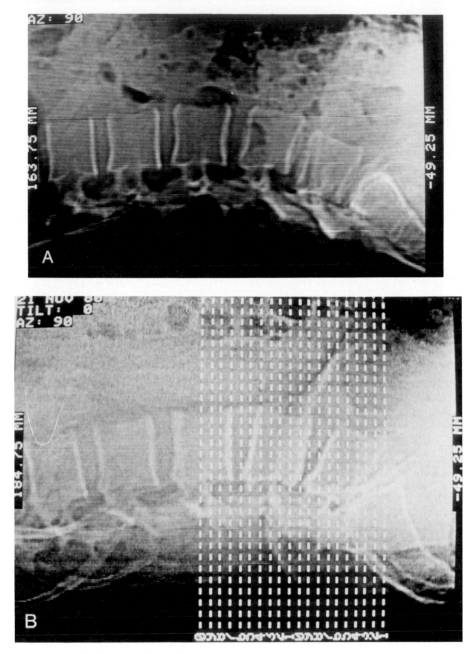

Figure 3.1.   A. Lateral localizing radiograph of the lumbar spine shows degenerative disc disease at L4–5 with grade I degenerative spondylolisthesis. The computed radiograph is used to determine the location of the actual scans. In the absence of scoliosis, excellent true lateral views of the intervertebral discs are obtained. B. The *numbered dashed lines*, representing the level of the obtained 5-mm contiguous slices, are placed on the computed radiograph following completion of the CT spine scan. C. Midsagittal reformatted image demonstrates the Grade I spondylolisthesis and build-up of the disc posteriorly at the level of the slip (*arrow*). D. Axial radiograph at the level of the slip demonstrates prominent L4–5 disc, marked degenerative changes in the posterior zygoapophyseal joints with ligamentous thickening, and severe central stenosis.

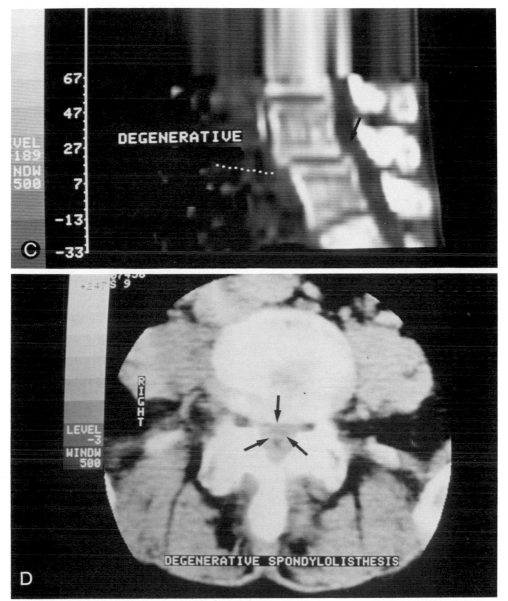

Figure 3.1 C and D.

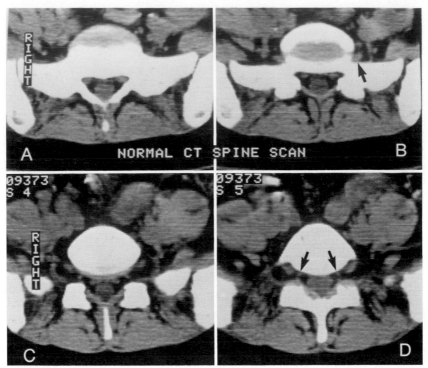

Figure 3.2.   Normal sequential axial CT scans from S1 through L4 are shown. A. A scan through S1 shows the S1 nerve roots and the thecal sac. Normal epidural veins lie between the vertebral body and the thecal sac. B. Inferior L5-S1 level with ligamentum flavum form the posterior aspect of the central canal. The normal S1 nerve roots lie in the subarticular recesses. The L5 nerve roots have exited the L5-S1 nerve root canal and lie on the anterior aspect of the sacrum adjacent the disc space (*arrow*). C. L5-S1 nerve root canal: the S1 nerve roots have just emerged from the anterolateral aspect of the thecal sac. They lie adjacent to the normal thin rim of L5-S1 disc seen posterior to the L5 vertebral body. The anterior internal vertebral veins lie within the nerve root canal. The L5 nerve roots lie at the foramen. The abundant epidural fat in the central canal and nerve root canals contrast sharply with these normal structures of higher density. D. Superior aspect of the L5-S1 nerve root canal showing the L5 nerve root ganglia at the foramen of the nerve root canal. The anterior internal vertebral veins are demonstrated as punctate densities within the medial aspect of the nerve root canal (*arrow*). E. Inferior aspect of L5 with prominent trefoil configuration of the lumbar spine. The lateral recesses are not sharply angled, however, and the L5 nerve roots are not compressed. Anastomosing epidural veins present as linear structures medial to the nerve roots and anterior to the thecal sac. F. Midbody of L5: note the triangular configuration of the canal, and the nerve roots within the lateral recess. G. Superior aspect of L5: this is the inferior aspect of the L4–5 interosseous segment and the posterior aspect of the canal is formed by ligamentum flavum. H. L4–5 disc level: the apparent narrowing of the intervertebral nerve root canals is due to imaging immediately above the pedicle at the very inferior aspect of the nerve root canal which tapers normally as it approaches the pedicle. At this level, the L5 nerve roots are emerging from the anterolateral aspect of the thecal sac. I. Superior aspect of the L4–5 disc: the L4 nerve roots have emerged from the L4–5 foramina. Note the prominent anterior internal vertebral veins within the nerve root canals medial to the L4 nerve roots. J. L4–5 nerve root canals demonstrate the emerging L4 nerve roots and their radicular veins extend between the thecal sac and the exiting nerve roots. K. The level immediately below the pedicle demonstrates the L4 nerve root ganglia as rounded structures in the very superior medial aspect of the L4–5 nerve root canal. The anastomosing epidural veins are the linear structures lying between the nerve root and the thecal sac. L. The intraosseous segment of L4 is shown.

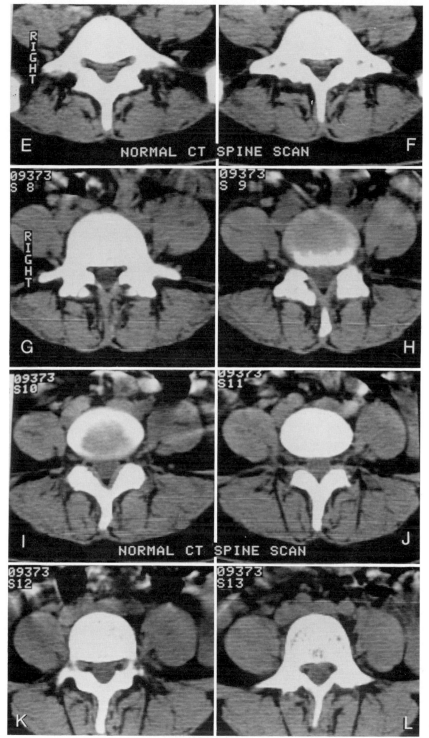

Figure 3.2 E–L.

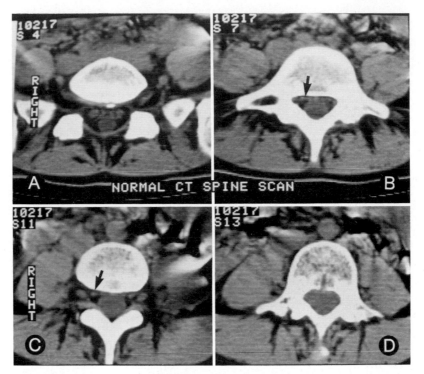

Figure 3.3.   This is a composite view of the L4–5 and L5-S1 nerve root canals and the intraosseous segments of L4 and 5. A. The S1 nerve roots are emerging from the anterior anterolateral aspect of the thecal sac. The comma-shaped structures lying between the thecal sac and the nerve roots represent epidural veins. The L5 nerve roots lie at the L5-S1 foramen. The normal S1 disc contains a small particle of calcification. Imaging of the disc posterior to the vertebral body of L5 is normal and due to angulation of the x-ray beam with respect to the disc space. Note the symmetry of the displayed disc. B. Intraosseous segment of L5: the L5 nerve roots lie in the subarticular gutter. The linear structure lying between the L5 nerve root and the thecal sac represents anastomotic venous channels between the AIVV (*arrow*). L4–5 nerve root canals with the L4 ganglia identified as rounded structures at the foramen of the nerve root canal are shown. The anterior internal vertebral vein (*arrow*) lies in intimate contact to the L4–5 disc and the medial aspect of the foramen and is approximately one-third of the size of the L4 nerve root ganglia. Note that the neural structures are well visualized because of the surrounding fat. Pathologic encroachment on the nerve root canal would obliterate the epidural fat. D. Interosseous segment of L4: note that there is no epidural fat and the entire central canal is normally filled with the thecal sac.

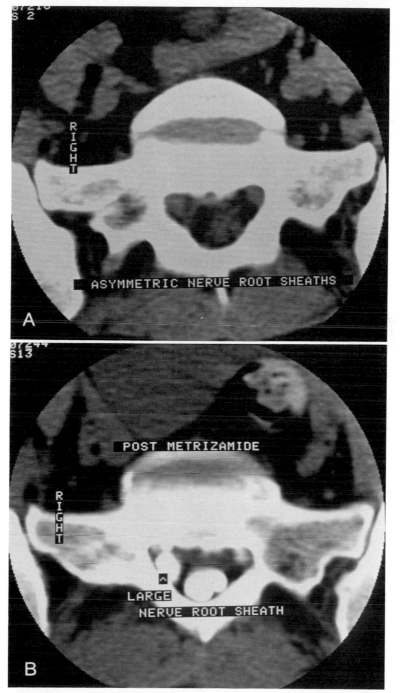

Figure 3.4.   Anatomic variation in nerve root sheaths is shown. A. Non-enhanced CT scan with asymmetry of the S1 nerve root is shown. No pathologic constricting lesion was identified and, therefore, this was presumed to represent an anatomic variant. B. Postmetrizamide CT scan confirms that the asymmetry is due to a large nerve root sheath.

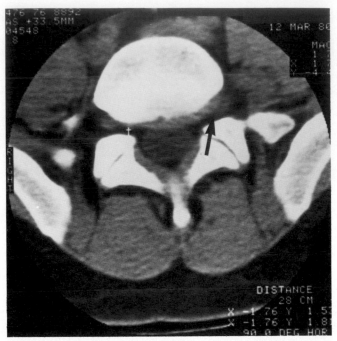

Figure 3.5. An asymmetric herniated L5-S1 disc is on the left. The L5 nerve root is displaced posterolaterally by the disc (*arrow*).

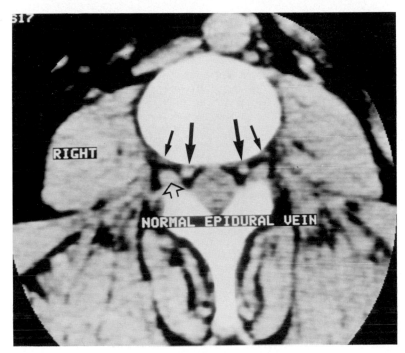

Figure 3.6. Normal anterior internal vertebral veins present as two paired veins on either side as in this case. The larger of the pair lies just medial to the nerve root ganglia (*large arrow*). The smaller of the paired veins lies at the foramen just ventral to the nerve root ganglia (*small arrows*). The nerve root ganglia (*open arrow*) lie ventral to the posterior zygoapophyseal joints. Fat surrounding the anterior aspect of the ganglia assures that no significant lateral entrapment is present.

38

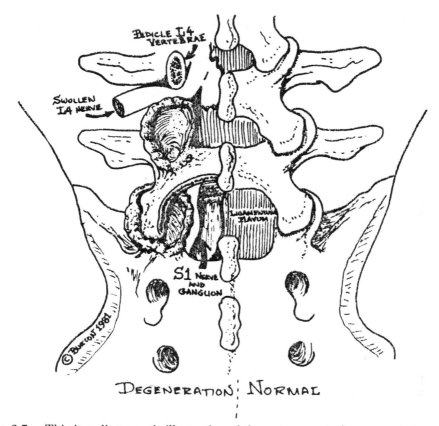

Figure 3.7.   This is a diagramatic illustration of the entrapment of nerve roots by spondylotic changes in the posterior element. The L4 nerve root is compressed by marked hypertrophic overgrowth of the superior articular process of L5 which results in entrapment of the nerve between the superior articular process and the pedicle. At the L5-S1 level, the nerve root is compressed in the subarticular recess by medial overgrowth of the superior articular process of S1. Most often, this hypertrophic change is seen in conjunction with a degenerative bulging disc. The S1 nerve root takes a rollercoaster course over the disc and under the superior articular process.

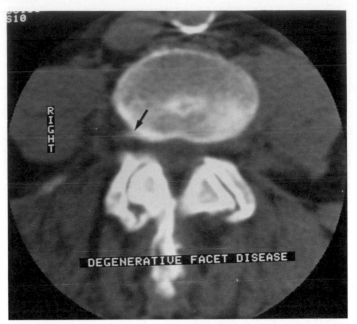

Figure 3.8. Marked degenerative disease of the zygoapophyseal joints is shown. There is severe erosion of the anterior aspect of the superior articular processes which, when severe, gives rise to degenerative spondylolisthesis. Note the posterior osteophyte on the right arising from the vertebral body which narrows the lateral aspect of the nerve root canal and indents the anterior aspect of the L4 nerve root ganglia (*arrow*).

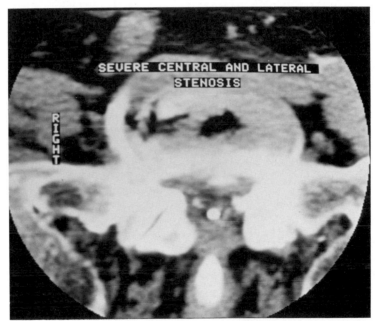

Figure 3.9. Severe degenerative disc disease is evidenced by fissuring of the disc and gas within the disc. There are marked hypertrophic changes involving the superior articular processes. There is also asymmetric bulging at the disc with disc density material filling the left subarticular gutter. A combination of degenerative disc disease and degenerative changes of the posterior elements leads to severe central spinal stenosis. Note droplets of pantopaque within the lumbar subarachnoid space.

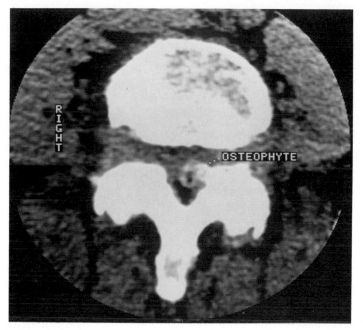

Figure 3.10.   Severe degenerative disease of the zygoapophyseal joints leads to production of large medially projecting osteophyte which encroaches significantly on the central canal.

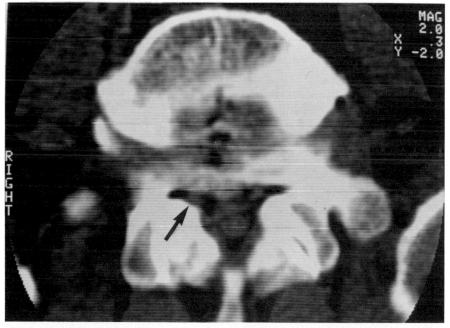

Figure 3.11.   Superior articular process (subarticular recess impingement) syndrome is demonstrated in this patient with severe degenerative disc disease and zygoapophyseal joint disease. The right S1 nerve root is trapped between the asymmetrically bulging disc and the hypertrophic superior articular facet (*arrow*). In our experience, the subarticular recess syndrome is most common at the L5-S1 level and, in most cases, the nerves are compressed in the subarticular recess by a combination of medial enlargement of the superior articular process and disc bulge or herniation.

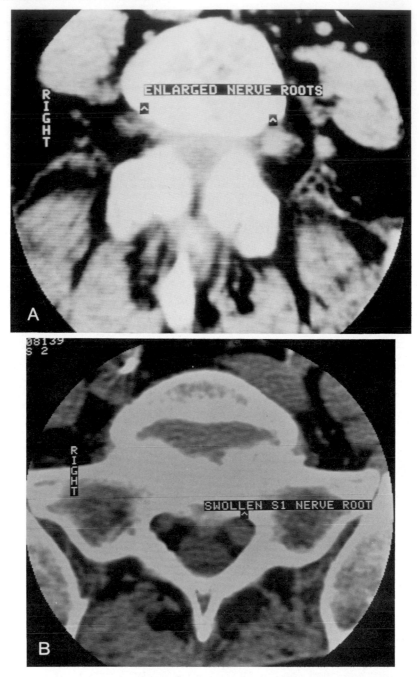

Figure 3.12. Enlarged nerve roots are demonstrated. A. There is bilateral pathologic enlargement of the L4 nerve roots as they emerge from the L4–5 nerve root canal. In this case, the enlargement was due to incorporation of the nerve roots within the fibrotic reaction at the margin of the L4–5 disc in degenerative spondylolisthesis. No lateral stenosis was present. B. Swollen left S1 nerve root secondary to poststenotic swelling due to a herniated disc which entrapped the S1 nerve root at a higher level.

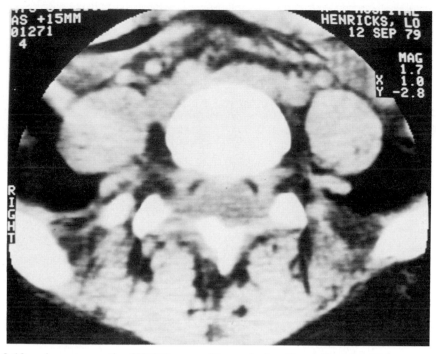

Figure 3.13.   A postoperative HRCT scan with marked epidural fibrosis which extends antero-laterally along the thecal sac and envelopes the exiting L5 nerve roots following posterior interbody fusion is shown.

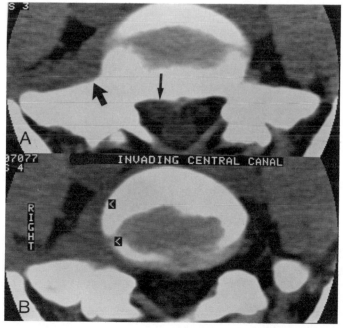

Figure 3.14.   Disc space infection is shown. A. Soft tissue retroperitoneal mass envelopes the L5 nerve root (*large arrow*). The S1 nerve root is considerably enlarged. B. Extension of the inflammatory process into the L5-S1 nerve root canal on the right is shown. There is direct extension into the central canal around the S1 nerve root and has caused enlargement of that nerve root.

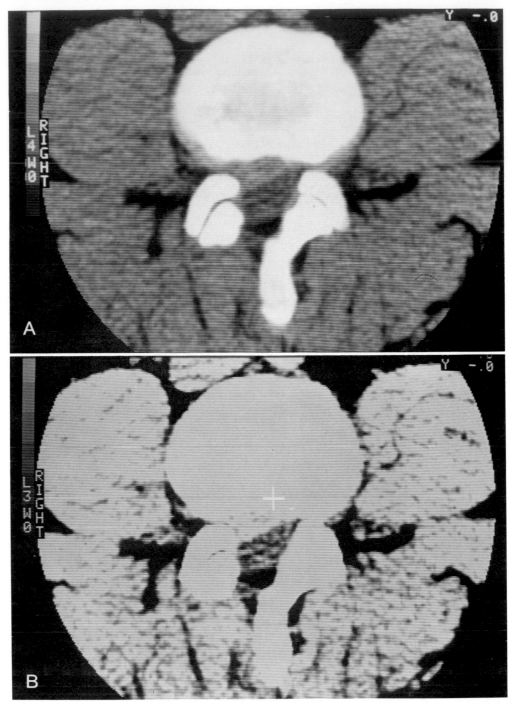

Figure 3.15. This is an illustration of the importance of a narrow window width in the visualization and diagnosis of disc disease. A. 1000 window width setting: A recurrent disc herniation is visualized, but poorly. B. A narrow window width improves the ability to visualize soft tissues such as discs. With this window setting, the recurrent herniated disc is well defined.

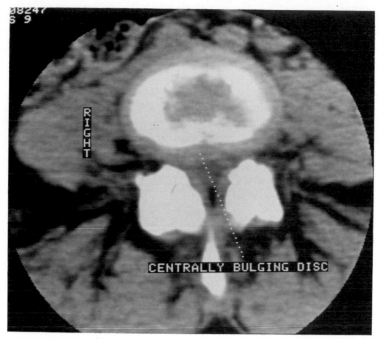

Figure 3.16. Degenerative disc disease L4–5 with a diffusely bulging disc annulus is shown. Associated degenerative disease of the posterior elements has caused overgrowth of the superior articular facets. There is central stenosis caused by this large centrally bulging disc and thickening of the ligamentum flavum.

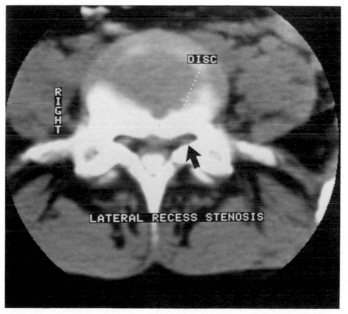

Figure 3.17. Marked narrowing of the left subarticular recess is demonstrated. This is caused by a combination of asymmetric bulging of the L4–5 disc and prominent medial hypertrophy of the superior articular facet and base of the lamina. The ganglion of the L5 nerve root is flattened between the disc and the superior articular process (*arrow*). The subarticular recess on the right is also somewhat narrowed. However, there is no disc bulge to compromise further the lateral recess and the nerve root ganglia on the right has a normal rounded configuration.

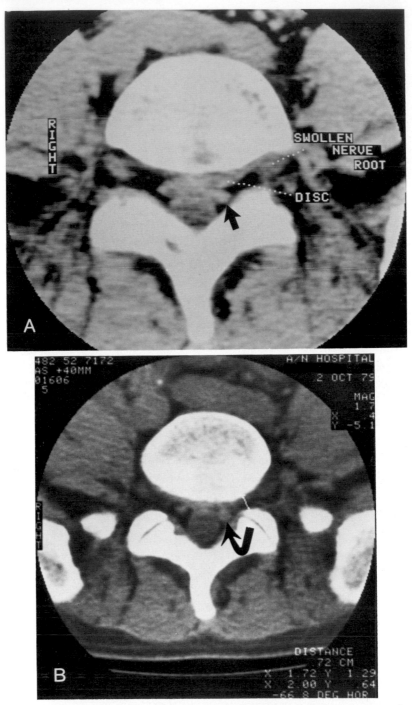

Figure 3.18.   Axial HRCT demonstrates a classical herniated disc on a non-enhanced HRCT scan. A. A herniated disc is imaged as a triangular high density structure which displaces the S1 nerve root posteriorly (*arrow*). B. A swollen S1 nerve root is immediately below the level of the herniated disc (*curved arrow*). Note a decreased amount of epidural fat, the indistinctness of the margin of the S1 nerve root, and the increased density of the fat due to edema of the nerve root and infiltration of the epidural fat.

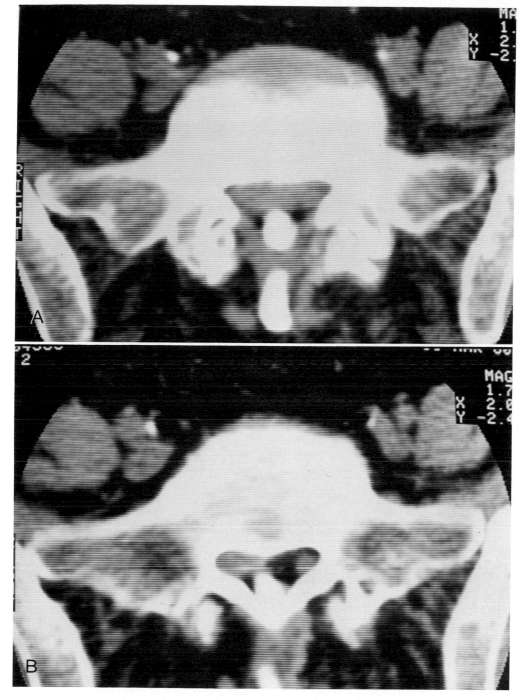

Figure 3.19. A. A huge centrally herniated disc fragment occupies the large epidural space between the vertebral body of S1 and the thecal sac. Because of this large space, this fragment causes little deformity of the thecal sac but does compress the S1 nerve roots bilaterally. B. Inferior extension of a large centrally herniated disc fragment into the right lateral recess with obliteration of the right S1 nerve root is shown.

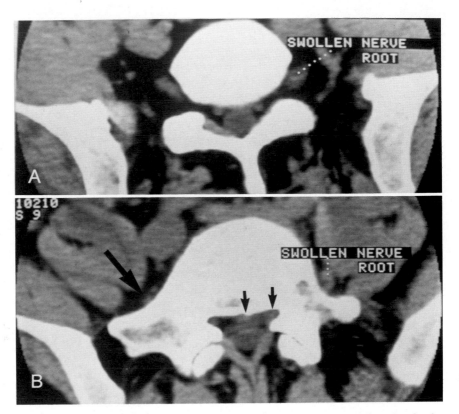

Figure 3.20. Axial HRCT image shows swelling of the L5 nerve root as it exits the foramen (A) and distally as it lies on the anterior aspect of the sacral ala. Note the asymmetry in the size of the nerve root when compared to its companion on the right (*large arrow*). Also, note soft disc herniation on the left at L5-S1 with compression of the left S1 nerve root and obliteration of the normal fat in the subarticular recess (*small arrow*).

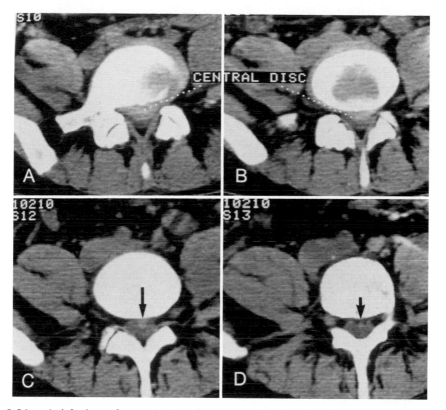

Figure 3.21. Axial views demonstrate a huge centrally herniated disc fragment. In A and B, marked compression of the thecal sac is shown. The disc fills the entire lateral recess on the left. The thecal sac is compressed to a small c-shaped structure on the right and posteriorly. C. The superior aspect of the disc herniation is demonstrated as a sharply angled free fragment which extends superiorly to lie posterior to the body of L4 (*arrow*). D. The very apex of the herniation strips the thecal sac away from the posterior aspect of the L4 vertebral body (*arrow*).

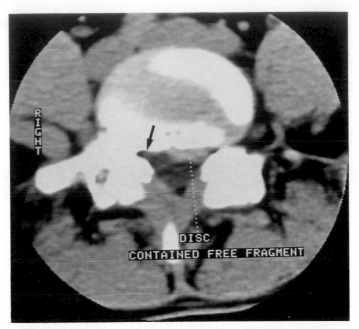

Figure 3.22. Axial image at the L4–5 level shows a squared off free fragment herniation which compresses the anterolateral aspect of the thecal sac on the left and obliterates the epidural fat in the lateral recess with compression of the L5 nerve root. At surgery, this was a free fragment herniation contained behind the posterior longitudinal ligament. Note the position of the normal L5 nerve root in the lateral recess on the right (*arrow*).

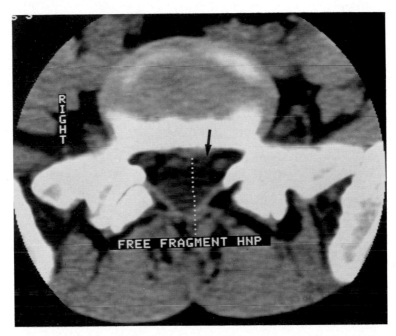

Figure 3.23. Axial image of the S1 vertebra immediately below the L5-S1 disc space shows the inferior aspect of a free fragment herniation. Note the asymmetry with flattening of the left anterolateral aspect of the thecal sac. Also, note posterior displacement of the epidural veins which lie between the thecal sac and the disc. The asymmetry of the disc protrusion plus the inferior migration to lie posterior to the S1 vertebral body are important signs of disc herniation on axial HRCT images.

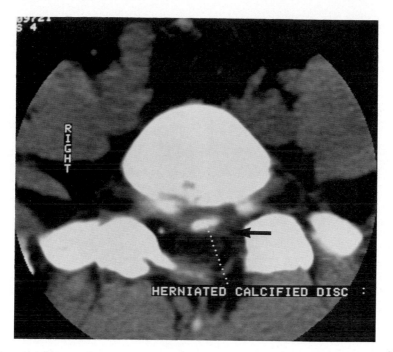

Figure 3.24. Axial image demonstrates asymmetric central and left-sided protrusion of a partially calcified herniated L5-S1 disc. Note the asymmetric flattening of the thecal sac and obliteration of a large portion of the epidural fat on the left by the herniated disc. The epidural vein on the left is flattened and displaced posteriorly (*arrow*). Note thickening of the ligamentum flavum posteriorly with irregular indentation of the posterior aspect of the thecal sac.

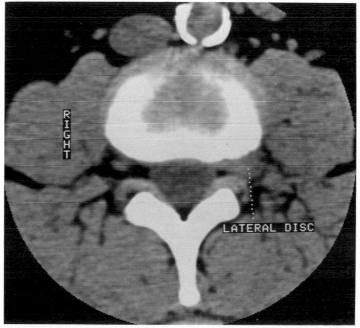

Figure 3.25. Axial image demonstrates a large lateral free disc fragment at the L3–4 level. Note obliteration of the normal epidural fat in the nerve root canal by the large, wedge-shaped, high density fragment. Also, the image of the L3 nerve root is completely lost because of compression and displacement. Note the absence of any deformity of the thecal sac by this laterally herniated disc. There is minimal symmetrical annular disc bulging.

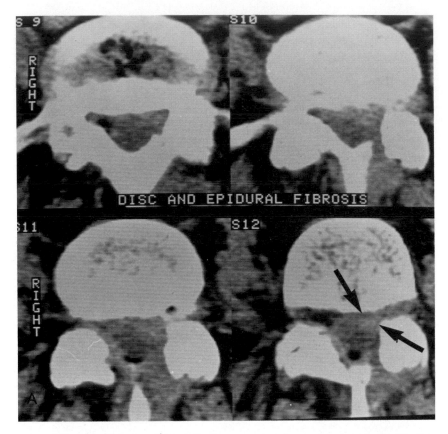

Figure 3.26. Recurrent herniated L4–5 disc in a previously operated patient with dense epidural fibrosis is shown. A. Axial images demonstrate extensive postoperative epidural fibrosis which extend into the central canal from the previous hemilaminotomy on the left. This extends anteriorly as a broad band of fibrosis to extend into both the exiting L4 nerve roots (*bottom right*) and the L5 nerve root in the lateral recess on the left (*top left*). Underlying the extensive and dense fibrosis is a recurrent free fragment disc herniation on the left. Differences in attenuation values between the disc and the epidural fibrosis were barely apparent using very narrow window settings to enhance the contrast and are very poorly discriminated on these images with a 250 window width. Note also the presence of residual postoperative lateral stenosis on the left due to a large posterior osteophyte and chronic disc protrusion. B. Measurement of the attentuation values of the scar and the recurrent disc, however, allowed confident diagnosis of the recurrent disc. The area under the square box (*thin arrow*) had a mean density of 121. This is compatible with a density of disc material showing attentuation values of the scar in the 70s and low 80s. The author has noted no epidural fibrosis with attenuation values above 90 (in patients who have not received intravenous contrast material) and most epidural fibrosis measures from 50–80 Hounsfield units.

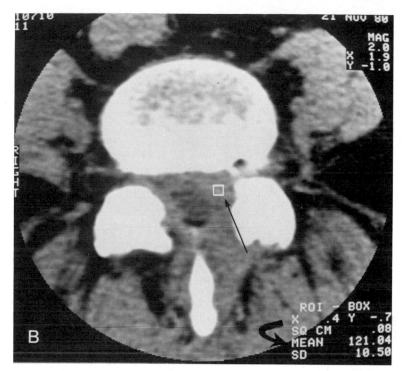

Figure 3.26. B.

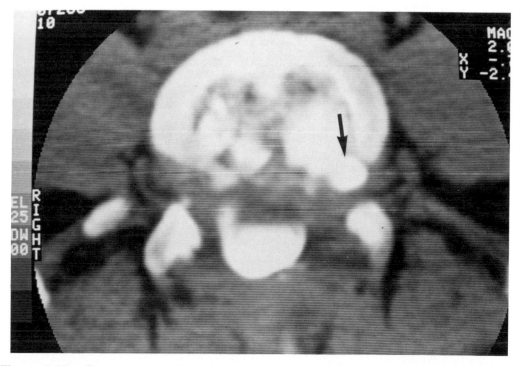

Figure 3.27. Transverse scan shows a posterior interbody fusion at L4–5 with posterior displacement of the bone plug causing lateral stenosis on the left. Note also the extensive epidural fibrosis which surrounds the thecal sac and extends into the nerve root canals bilaterally.

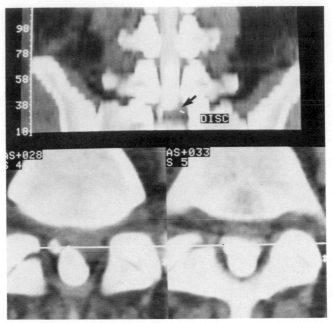

Figure 3.28. Postmetrizamide-enhanced transverse and coronal reformatted images of an acute herniated disc at L5-S1 are shown on the left. Note the direct imaging of the herniated disc material which flattens the anterolateral aspect of the thecal sac and compresses the left S1 nerve root; causing nonfilling of the nerve root sheath on the reformatted image (*arrow*). Note the obliteration of the normal epidural fat in the lateral recess.

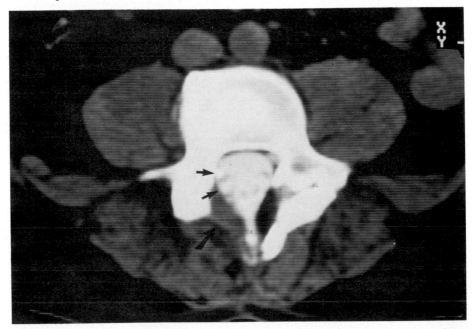

Figure 3.29. Transverse image shows a postoperative right L4 hemilaminectomy with postoperative epidural fibrosis and arachnoiditis. Note the epidural fibrosis in the posterolateral aspect of the canal on the right (*large arrow*) and associated irregularity of the margin of the thecal sac as well as thickening of the nerve roots lying adjacent the small droplets of pantopaque within the thecal sac (*small arrow*).

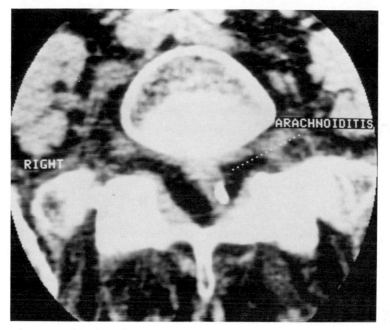

Figure 3.30. A transverse scan of the L5-S1 level in a patient with arachnoiditis documented at myelography is shown. Note the contraction of the thecal sac with an increase in the surrounding epidural fat in the dorsal lateral aspect of the central canal. Also note the dense residual droplet of pantopaque.

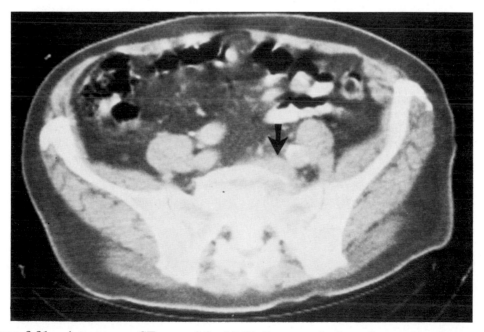

Figure 3.31. A transverse CT scan of the L5-S1 disc space is shown in a patient with discitis. Note the resorption of the bony margins of the disc on the left and the associated presacral, retroperitoneal soft tissue mass silhouetting the left iliac vein (*arrow*).

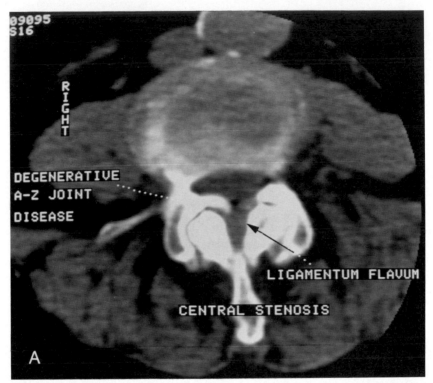

Figure 3.32. Transverse scans show degenerative zygoapophyseal joint disease. A. There is marked bony overgrowth and scalloping of the superior articular facets. The marked erosive changes cause both hypertrophy and marginal osteophyte formation which envelope the inferior articular facets. This was associated with marked loss of disc volume and bulging of the disc annulus. Note the thickening of the ligamentum flavum which fills the entire dorsolateral aspect of the central canal. The central canal also is encroached upon by the large osteophyte projecting medially from the right superior articular process. B. Marked asymmetry of the zygoapophyseal joints with a cup-shaped joint on the left and fragmentation of the zyogapophyseal joint on the right is shown. C. Widening of the anteromedial aspect of the zygoapophyseal joint space produces a clamshell appearance of the zygoapophyseal joint. Note narrowing of the posterolateral aspect of the joint space and fragmentation of the anteromedial aspect of the superior articular processes at the site of attachment of the ligamentum flavum. The ligamentum flavum and joint capsule stretch across the gaping facet joint on the left (*arrow*).

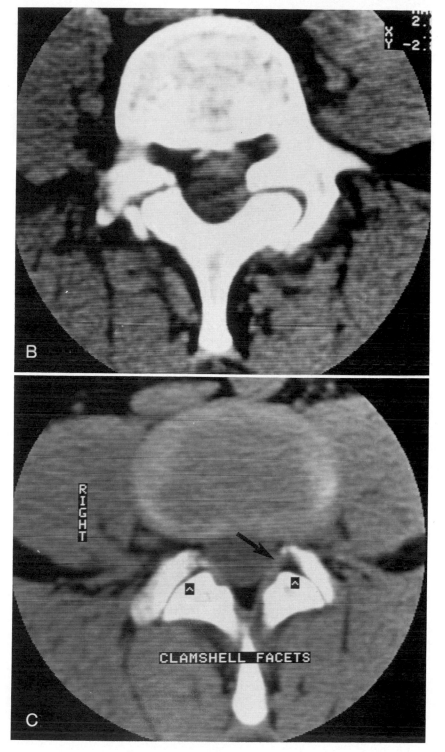

Figure 3.32. B and C.

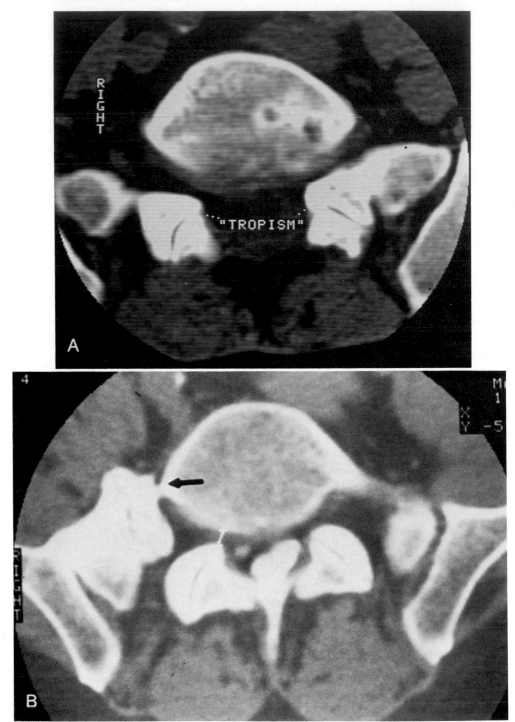

Figure 3.33.   Transverse scans of L5-S1 demonstrating tropism or asymmetry of the zygoapophyseal joints. A. Note the asymmetry of the orientation of the zygoapophyseal joints with an abnormal sagittal orientation of the right L5-S1 zygoapophyseal joint. This is an unstable orientation and may predispose to rotational instability. B. Tropism of the posterior zygoapophyseal joints at L5-S1 and partial sacralization of L5 on the right with a pseudojoint formation (*arrow*) is shown.

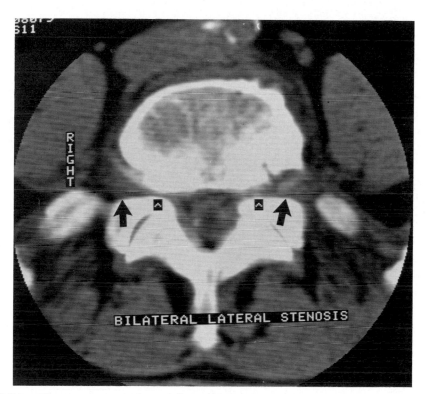

Figure 3.34.   Transverse scan shows bilateral lateral stenosis at the L4–5 level. Note marked narrowing of both lateral nerve root canals caused by a combination of large posterolateral osteophytes arising from the margin of the L5 vertebral body and concomitant hypertrophic overgrowth of the superior articular processes. Both L4 nerve roots are swollen as they exit the narrowed foramen (*arrow*).

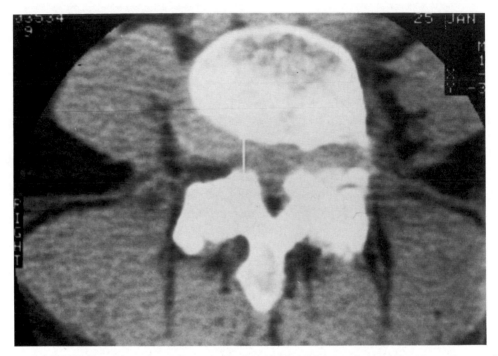

Figure 3.35. Transverse scans show marked central and lateral stenosis. Note the marked hypertrophic overgrowth of the zygoapophyseal joints with fragmentation of the zygoapophyseal joint on the left. The lateral stenosis is caused by marked posterior bulging of the L4–5 disc which fills the entire canal on the left and bulges far posteriorly on the right. The bony nerve root canal on the right is normal. On the left, the canal is elongated and narrowed by both the bony fragmentation of the hypertrophic superior articular process of L5 and a large square osteophyte arising from the vertebral body. Hypertrophic overgrowth of the left inferior articular facet encroaches on the dorsolateral aspect of the central canal and indents the thecal sac.

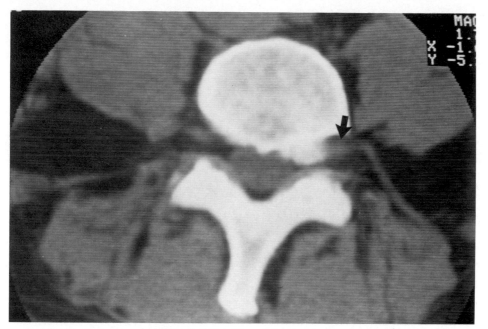

Figure 3.36. Transverse scans show left L4–5 lateral stenosis caused by a large focal osteophyte arising from the posterolateral aspect of the vertebral body. There is enlargement and lateral displacement of the exiting L4 nerve root (*arrow*). Compare with the normal right L4–5 nerve root canal and exiting L4 nerve root.

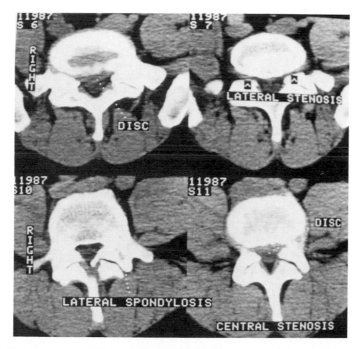

Figure 3.37. Transverse scan shows advanced multilevel central and lateral spinal stenosis. Note a centrally herniated L5-S1 disc (*upper left*), as well as severe bilateral lateral stenosis at L5-S1 (*upper right*). At the L4–5 level (*lower right*), there is compromise of the central canal caused by a combination of centrally bulging disc and hypertrophic changes of the superior and inferior articular facets.

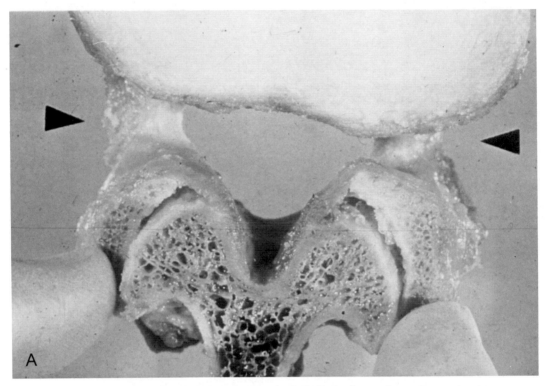

Figure 3.38. Dynamic lateral stenosis is shown. A. Pathologic specimen demonstrating narrowing of the left L4–5 nerve root canal by rotation of the specimen, such that the superior articular facet of L5 rotates anteriorly toward the intervertebral disc and vertebral body of L4. Note widening of the ipsilateral zygoapophyseal joint space and stretching of the ligamentum flavum. B. Transverse CT scan produced in extension and rotation. Patient's shoulders were flat on the table and the left hip was elevated. Note flattening of the posterior aspect of the left L4–5 nerve root ganglion by the superior articular facet (*arrow*). Note also the normal oval appearance of the right nerve root ganglion (*upper right*). Note slight widening of the left L4–5 zygoapophyseal joint (*upper left*). C. Right anterior oblique transverse scans at the L4–5 level are shown. Note in this rotation that the posterior aspect of the left L4 nerve root ganglion is no longer imprinted by the superior articular process and that now the posterior aspect of the right L4–5 ganglion is indented by the superior articular process (*arrow*). This sequence demonstrates that slight dynamic movement of the superior articular process can produce critical narrowing of borderline nerve root canals with resultant impingement on the nerve root ganglia.

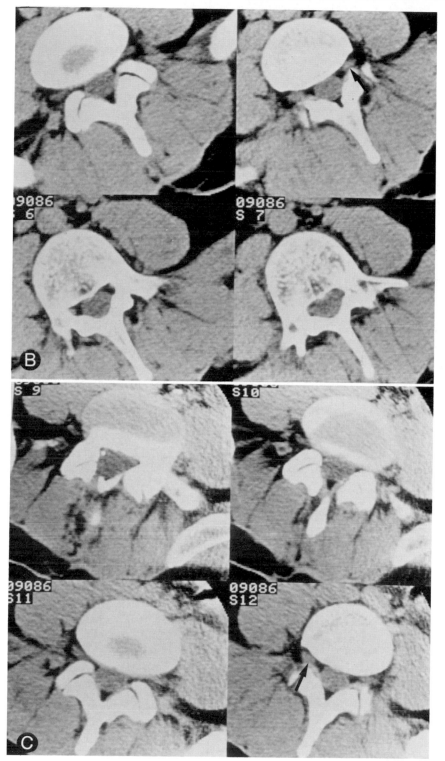

Figure 3.38. B and C.

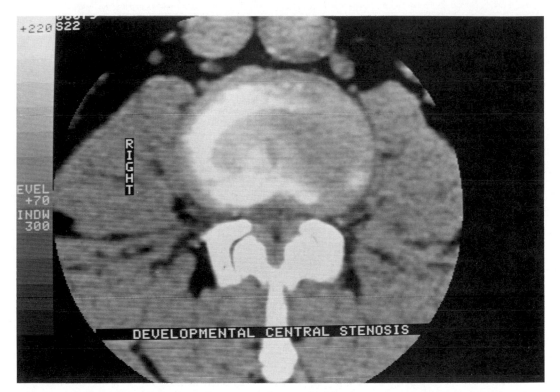

Figure 3.39. Transverse scans show central stenosis. The bony measurements of the canal are decreased. There are superimposed degenerative changes of diffuse annular bulging of the disc as well as hypetrophic changes of the superior and inferior articular facets and thickening of the ligamentum flavum. At this stage, it is difficult to decide whether the stenosis is developmental or degenerative in nature. In this patient, the sagittal measurements were diminished throughout the lumbosacral spine and this is presumed to be developmental in origin.

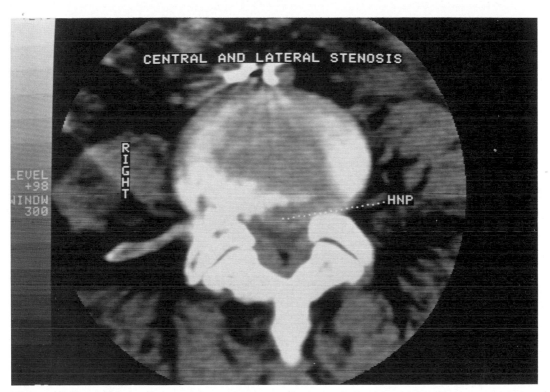

Figure 3.40. Transverse scan shows severe central stenosis in a patient with degenerative central and lateral spinal stenosis. Note the centrally protruding disc which is asymmetrical and more prominent on the left than on the right. There are associated degenerative changes in posterior zygoapophyseal joints with considerable hypertrophy of the superior and inferior articular facets and thickening of the lamina. The ligamentum flavum is also thickened. The central canal is markedly narrowed with a triangular outwardly concave appearance. The bulging disc completely fills the left L4–5 subarticular gutter and compression of the L5 nerve root by the disc was present at surgery.

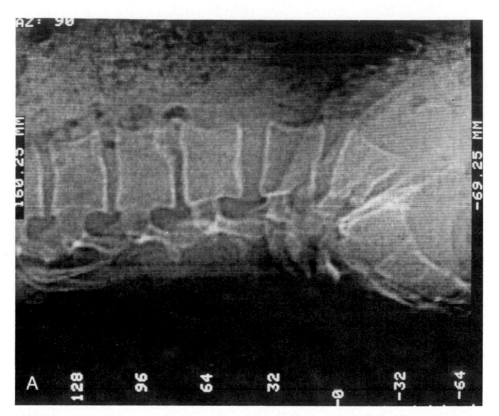

Figure 3.41. Grade II spondylolytic spondylolisthesis at L5-S1 is shown. A. Computed radiograph shows Grade II spondylolisthesis of L5 on S1. There is marked narrowing of the posterior aspect of the disc space as well as anteroinferior displacement of L5 on S1. B. Transverse scans of the L5-S1 level: because of the anterior and inferior slippage of L5 on S1, the disc is imaged as a transverse low density bar between the L5 vertebral body and S1 (*upper left and upper right*). Note the appearance of the thecal sac at the site of the emergence of the S1 nerve roots (*upper right*) within the sacral canal on the scan immediately below. The spondylolytic break in the pars interarticularis of L5 is shown well (*lower right*). There is bilateral entrapment of the exiting L5 nerve roots caused by the anterior and inferior slippage of the pars superior to lie within the nerve root canal. This is demonstrated well on the right (*lower left*). The L5 nerve roots are compressed between the centrally prominent L5-S1 disc anteriorly and inferiorly (*broad arrow on the lower right*), and the hypertrophied pars posteriorly and superiorly (*lower left*). Note the marked poststenotic swelling of the L5 nerve roots (*arrows, lower left*). These L5 nerve roots are also compressed within the nerve root canal (*arrows, upper right*) and as they exit the flattened L5-S1 neural foramina (*arrows, upper left*). C. Sagittal reformatted image demonstrating the anterior slippage of L5 on S1 as well as the posterior prominence of the L5-S1 disc.

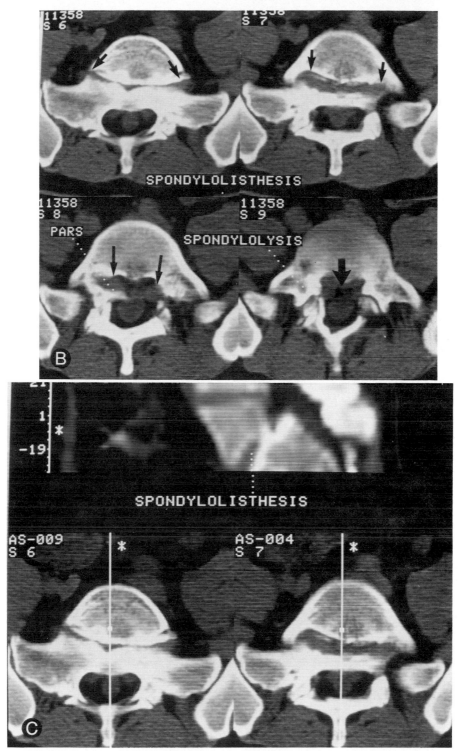

Figure 3.41. B and C.

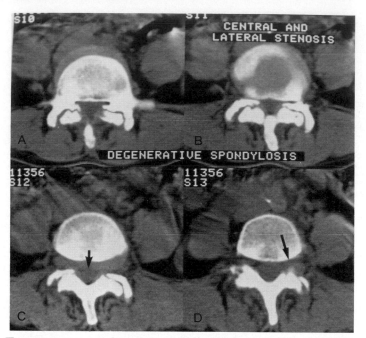

Figure 3.42. Transverse scans show severe degenerative spondylosis of the zygoapophyseal joints with resultant degenerative spondylolisthesis. The marked erosion of these superior articular processes allows anterior slippage of the L4 vertebral body on L5. Note the marked cupping of the superior articular processes and fraying and irregularity of the zygoapophyseal joints. The posterior prominence of the disc (*lower left*) is caused by anterior slippage of the entire L4 vertebral body on L5 with resultant anterior movement of the inferior articular facets and lamina to impinge on the disc and nerve root canals. There is associated degenerative narrowing of the disc space and, consequently, of the nerve root canals. There is severe lateral stenosis on the left with entrapment of the exiting L4 nerve root between the prominent posterior bulging disc and the anteriorly displaced inferior articular facet (*arrow, lower right*). Anterior movement of the lamina and inferior articular facet and the posterior prominence of the disc cause central stenosis (*lower left*).

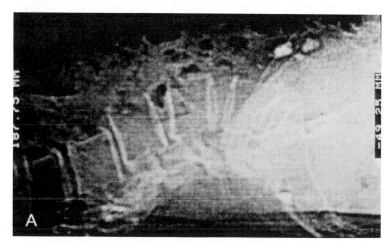

Figure 3.43. Retrospondylolisthesis: A. Computed radiograph demonstrates exaggerated lumbar lordosis and retrospondylolisthesis at L2–3 and L3–4.

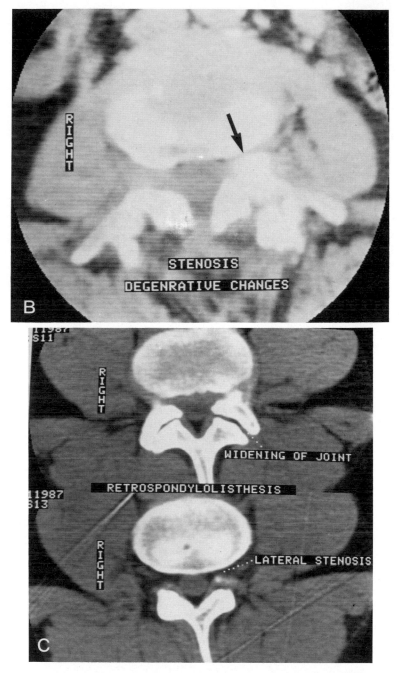

Figure 3.43. B. Transverse scan of the same patient at the L2–3 level demonstrates severe fragmenting of the posterior zygoapophyseal joints with marked lateral stenosis caused by posterior displacement of the L2 vertebral body against the hypertrophied and degenerated superior articular facet of L3 (*arrow*). C. Retrospondylolisthesis at the L3–4 level in the second patient shows widening of the zygoapophyseal joints and production of lateral spinal stenosis at L3–4 on the left due to posterior movement of the entire L3 vertebral body with respect to the superior articular process of L4.

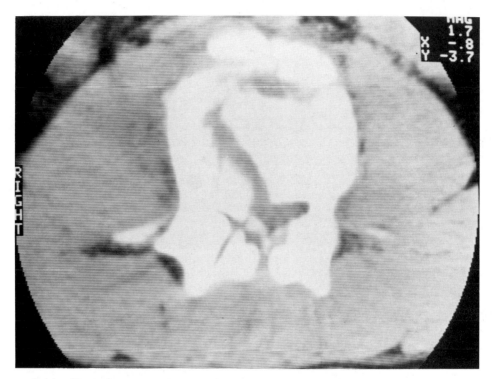

Figure 3.44. Transverse scan shows a severe burst fracture of L1 with marked deformity of the central spinal canal and displacement of two fragments into the canal.

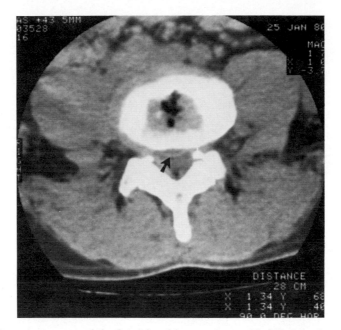

Figure 3.45. Transverse scan of the L4–5 level in a patient with failed back surgery syndrome is shown. The patient had had an L4–5 discectomy 14 months prior, with recurrence of back pain. The CT scan demonstrated developmental spinal stenosis with a recurrent central disc bulge (*arrow*) which contributed to the central stenosis. The patient also had annular bulging of the disc and bilateral lateral stenosis at the L4–5 level. No CT scan was done prior to the first surgical procedure and the central and lateral stenosis were unrecognized.

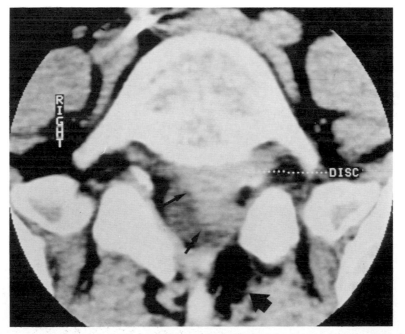

Figure 3.46. Transverse scan of the L5-S1 level of a failed back surgery syndrome patient is shown. Note the huge recurrent disc herniation on the left with marked compression of the thecal sac (*arrows*). Note the absent ligamentum flavum at the site of the previous hemilaminectomy and placement of a free fat graft (*broad arrow*). Note the lack of epidural fibrosis.

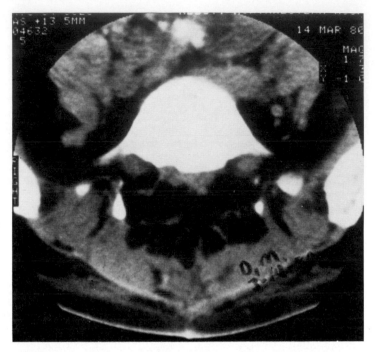

Figure 3.47. Transverse scan of the L5-S1 level in a patient with a complete posterior laminectomy and facetectomy is shown. Note the placement of the large epidural fat graft with compression of the thecal sac. The L5 nerve roots are completely surrounded by this fat graft and there is no evidence of postoperative epidural or perineural fibrosis.

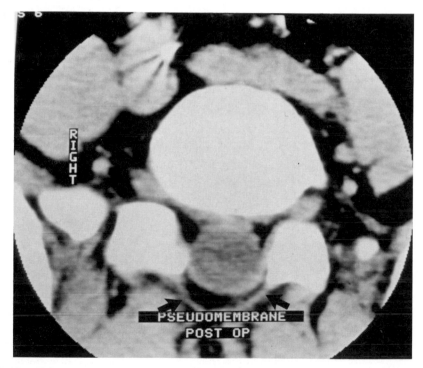

Figure 3.48. Transverse scan of the L5-S1 level is shown in a patient with postoperative decompressive laminectomy and fat grafting. Note the absence of epidural fibrosis and the presence of a pseudomembrane forming posterior to the fat graft (*arrows*).

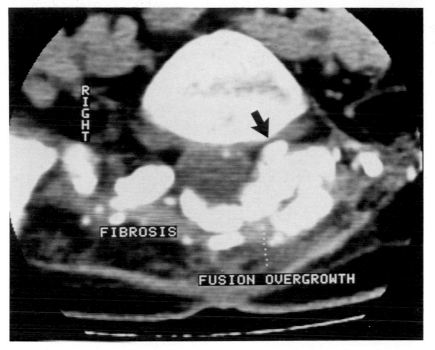

Figure 3.49.   Transverse scan of the L5-S1 level in a patient with previous laminectomy fusion shows marked fusion overgrowth with production of severe lateral stenosis at L5-S1 on the left (*arrow*).

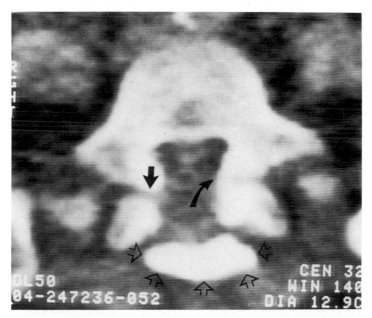

Figure 3.50.   Transverse scan of L5-S1 is shown in a patient with spondylolytic spondylolisthesis of L5. Note the break in the pars of L5 on the right (*broad arrow*) and spontaneous fusion of the break in the pars on the left (*curved arrow*). Note the failure of fusion of the posterior fusion bone to L5 (*open arrowhead*). The fusion extended from S1-L4. The fusion was solid at L4 and S1, but bridged the L5 vertebral body without fusing it. At surgery, there was motion on the right as predicted by the CT scan.

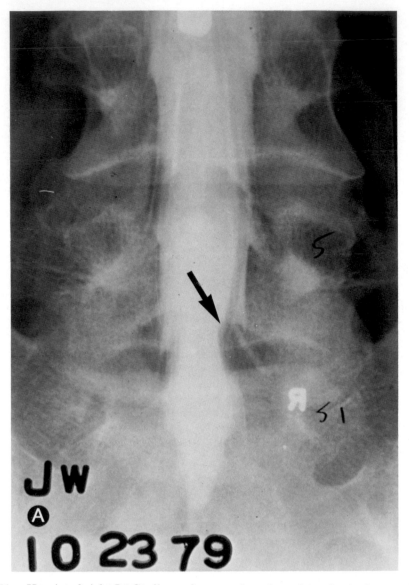

Figure 3.51. Herniated right L5-S1 disc and concomitant bony lateral spinal stenosis L5-S1 on the right. A. Posterior-anterior view of the metrizamide myelogram shows an extradural defect consistent with a classical herniated disc (*arrow*). Note displacement of the S1 nerve root. B. Transverse scan of a metrizamide-enhanced CT scan shows a classical triangular high density disc in the subarticular recess on the right with flattening of the thecal sac and obliteration of the S1 nerve root (*arrow*). Note also severe lateral spinal stenosis on the right due to marked hypertrophy of the superior articular process and a posterolateral osteophyte which causes squaring of the vertebral body (*curved arrow*). C. Immediate postoperative scan shows wide compressive laminectomy and placement of a large free fat graft with deformity of the thecal sac by the fat graft. There has been resection of a portion of the vertebral end plate at discectomy. Note relief of the lateral stenosis on the right side secondary to resection of the osteophyte, and more importantly, resection of the medial third of the superior articular facet. The soft tissue within the nerve root canal probably represents hemorrhage. There is a small bubble of air lying between the vertebral body and the soft tissue (*small arrow*).

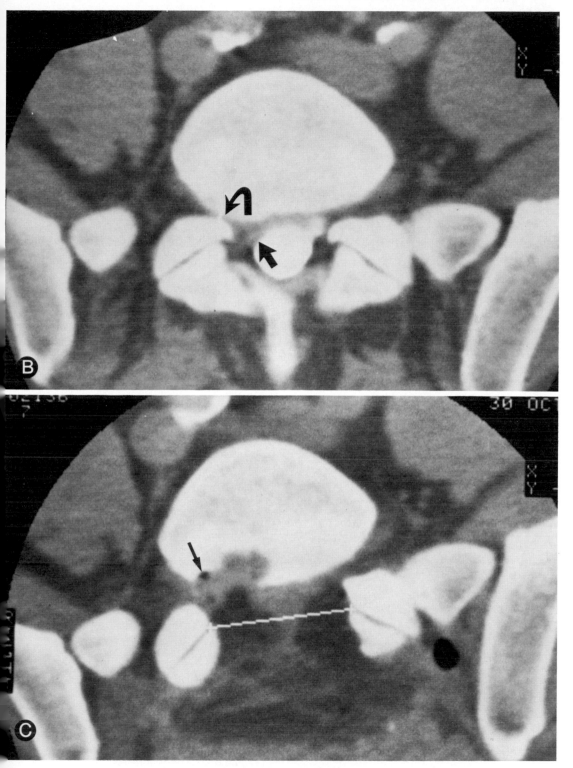

Figure 3.51. B and C.

76 LUMBAR SPINE SURGERY

References

1. Glenn, W. V., Davis, K. R., Dwyer, S. J.: Alternative display formats for computed tomography (CT) data. In: Current Concepts in Radiology, Vol. 3, edited by E. J. Potchen. St. Louis, CV Mosby Company, 1977.
2. Glenn, W. V., Johnston, R. J., Morton, P. E., Dwyer, S. J.: Further investigation and initial clinical use of advanced CT display capability. *Invest. Radiol. 10:* 479–489, 1975.
3. Glenn, W. V., Johnston, R. J., Morton, P. E., Dwyer, S. J.: Image generation and display techniques for CT scan data: thin transverse and reconstructed coronal and sagittal planes. *Invest. Radiol. 10:* 403–416, 1975.
4. Glenn, W. V., Lancourt, J. E., Wiltse, L. L.: Multiplanar CT applications in the spine: Early clinical experience. Proceedings of CT Conference, edited by M. Korobkin. San Francisco, University of California, 1978.
5. Glenn, W. V., Rhodes, M. L., Atlschuler, E. M., Wiltse, L. L., Kostanek, D., Kuo, Y. M.: Multiplanar display computed body tomography applications in the lumbar spine. *Spine 4:* 282–352, 1979.
6. Lancourt, J. E., Glenn, W. V., Wiltse, L. L.: Multiplanar computerized tomography in the normal spine and in the diagnosis of spinal stenosis: A gross anatomic-computerized tomographic correlation. *Spine 4:* 379–390, 1979.
7. Burton, C. V., Heithoff, K., Kirkaldy-Willis, W., Ray, C. D.: Computed tomographic Scanning and the lumbar spine. *Spine 4:* 356–368, 1979.
8. Gargano, F. P., Jacobson, R., Rosomoff, H.: Transverse axial tomography of the spine. *Neuroradiology 6:* 254–258, 1974.
9. Gargano, F. P., Jacobson, R.: Transverse axial tomography of the spine: Part III, the lumbar spine. *CRC Crit. Rev. Clin. Radiol. Nuclear Med. 8:* 311–328, 1976.
10. Hammerschlag, S. B., Wolpert, S. M., Carter, B. L.: Computed tomography of the spinal canal. *Radiology 121:* 361–367, 1976.
11. Isherwood, I., Fawcitt, R. A., Nettle, J. R. L., Spencer, J. W., Pullan, B. R.: Computed tomography of the spine: A preliminary report. In: Computerized Axial Tomography in Clinical Practice, edited by G. H. du Boulay, I. F. Moseley. Berlin, Springer Verlag, 1977, pp. 322–335.
12. Jacobson, R. E., Gargano, F. P., Rosomoff, H. L.: Transverse axial tomography of the spine, Parts 1 and 2. *J. Neurosurg. 42:* 406–419, 1975.
13. Lee, B. C. P., Kazam, E., Newman, A. P.: Computed tomography of the spine and spinal cord. *Radiology 128:* 95–102, 1978.
14. Sheldon, J. J., Sersland, T., Leborgne, J.: Computed tomography of the lower lumbar vertebral column. *Radiology 124:* 113–118, 1977.
15. Ullrich, C. G., Binet, E. F., Sanecki, M. G., Kieffer, S. A.: Quantitative assessment of the lumbar spinal canal by computed tomography. *Radiology 134:* 137–143, 1980.
16. Choudhury, A. R., Taylor, J. C.: Occult lumbar spinal stenosis. *J. Neurol. Neurosurg. Psychiatr. 40:* 506–510, 1977.
17. Coin, C. G., Chan, Y. S., Keranen, V., Pennink, M.: Computer assisted myelography in disc disease. *J. Comput. Assist. Tomogr. 1:* 398–404, 1977.
18. de Chiro, G., Schellinger, C.: Computed tomography of spinal cord after lumbar intrathecal introduction of metrizamide (computer assisted myelography). *Radiology 120:* 101–104, 1976.
19. Meyer, G. A., Haughton, V. M., Williams, A. L.: Diagnosis of herniated lumbar disc with computed tomography. *N. Engl. J. Med. 301:* 1166–1167, 1979.
20. Naidich, T. P., King, D. G., Moran, C. J., Sagel, S. S.: Computed tomography of the lumbar thecal sac. *J. Comput. Assist. Tomogr. 4:* 37–41, 1980.
21. Ciric, I., Mikhael, M. A., Tarkington, J. A., Vick, N. A.: The lateral recess syndrome: A variant of spinal stenosis. *J. Neurosurg. 53:* 433–445, 1980.
22. Epstein, J. A., Epstein, B. S., Rosenthal, A. D., Carras, R., Lavine, L. S.: Sciatica caused by nerve root entrapment in the lateral recess: The superior facet syndrome. *J. Neurosurg. 36:* 584–489, 1972.
23. Schlesinger, P. T.: Incarceration of the first sacral nerve in a lateral bony recess of the spinal canal as a cause of sciatica. *J. Bone Joint Surg. 37A:* 115, 1955.
24. Schlesinger, P. T.: Low lumbar nerve root compression and adequate operative exposure. *J. Bone Joint Surg. 39A:* 541, 1957.
25. Post, M. J. D.: Radiographic Evaluation of the Spine: Current Advances with Emphasis on Computed Tomography. Masson Publishing USA, Inc., New York, 1980.
26. McNabb, I.: Negative disc exploration: An analysis of the causes of nerve root involvement in sixty-eight patients. *J. Bone Joint Surg. 52:* 891–903, 1971.
27. Mixter, W. J., Barr, J. S.: Rupture of the intervertebral disc with involvement of the spinal canal. *N. Engl. J. Med. 211:* 210–215, 1934.
28. Harris, R. I., McNabb, I: Structural changes in the intervertebral disc. *J. Bone Joint Surg. 36B:* 304, 1954.
29. Hirsch, C., Schajowicz, FL: Studies on structural changes in the lumbar annulus fibrosus. *Acta Orthop. Scand. 22:* 184, 1953.
30. Richie, J. H., Fahrni, W. H.: Age changes in lumbar intervertebral discs. *Can. J. Surg. 13:* 65, 1970.
31. Yong-Hing, K., Reilly, J., Kirkaldy-Willis, W. H.: The ligamentum flavum. *Spine 1:* 226, 1976.
32. Benoist, M., Ficat, C., Baraf, P., Caudroix, J.: Postoperative lumbar epiduro-arachnoiditis: Diagnostic and therapeutic aspects. *Spine 5:* 432–436, 1980.
33. Burton, C. V., Wiltse, L. L.: Editorial Comment. *Spine 3:* 23, 1978.
34. Burton, C. V., Wiltse, L. L.: Editorial and symposium on lumbar arachnoiditis: Nomenclature, etiology and pathology. *Spine 3:* 23–92, 1978.
35. Burton, C. V., Kirkaldy-Willis, W., Yong-Hing, K., Heithoff, K. B.: Causes of failure of surgery on the lumbar spine. *Clin. Orthop. 157:* 191–199, 1981.
36. Crock, H. V.: A reappraisal of intervertebral disc lesions. *Med. J. Australia 1:* 983, 1970.
37. Farfan, H. F.: Effects of torsion on the intervertebral joints. *Can. J. Surg. 12:* 336, 1969.

38. Farfan, H. F.: Mechanical disorders of the low back. Lea & and Febiger, 1973.

39. Farfan, H. F.: The pathological anatomy of degenerative spondylolisthesis: A cadaver study. *Spine* 5:412–418, 1980.

40. Farfan, H. F., Sullivan, J. D.: The relation of facet orientation to intervertebral disc failure. *Can. J. Surg. 10:*179, 1967.

41. Kirkaldy-Willis, W. H., Heithoff, K. B., Bowen, C. V. A., Shannon, R.: Pathological anatomy of lumbar spondylosis and stenosis, correlated with the C.T. scan, radiographic evaluation of the spine. In: Current Advances with Emphasis on Computed Tomography, edited by M. J. D. Post. Masson Publishing, Inc., New York, 1980, pp. 34–55.

42. Kirkaldy-Willis, W. H., McIvor, G. W. D.: Spinal Stenosis. *Clin. Orthop. 115:*2–144, 1976.

43. Kirkaldy-Willis, W. H., Paine, K. W. E., Cauchoix, J., et al.: Lumbar spinal stenosis. *Clin. Orthop.* 99:30–50, 1974.

44. Kirkaldy-Willis, W. H., Wedge, J. H., Yong-Hing, K., Reilly, J.: Pathology and pathogenesis of lumbar spondylosis and stenosis. *Spine 3:*319–328, 1978.

45. Keim, H. A., Kirkaldy-Willis, W. H.: Low Back Pain. Clinical Symposia, Volume 32, No. 6, 1980 published by Ciba Pharmaceutical Co., Summit, NJ.

46. Keller, J. T., Dunsker, S. B., McWhorter, J. M., Ongkiko, C. M., Saunders, M. C., Mayfield, F. H.: The fate of autogenous grafts to the spinal dura. *J. Neurosurg. 49:*412–418, 1978.

47. Kestler, O. C.: Overgrowth (hypertrophy) of lumbosacral grafts causing a complete block. *Bull. Hosp. Joint Dis. 27:*51–57, 1966.

48. Crock, H. V.: Isolated lumbar disc resorption as a cause of nerve root canal stenosis. *Clin. Orthop. 115:*109, 1976.

49. Carrera, G. F., Haughton, V. M., Syvertsen, A., Williams, A. L.: Computed tomography of the lumbar facet joints. *Radiology 134:*145–148, 1980.

50. Williams, P. C.: Lumbar spine, reduced lumbosacral joint space. Its relation to sciatic irritation. *J.A.M.A. 99A:*1677, 1932.

51. Nelson, M. A.: Lumbar spinal stenosis. *J. Bone Joint Surg. 55:*506–512, 1973.

52. Post, M. J. D., Gargano, F. P., Vining, D. Q., Rosomoff, H. L.: A comparison of radiographic methods of diagnosing constrictive lesions of the spinal canal (Toshiba unit versus C. T. scanner). *J. Neurosurg. 48:*360–368, 1978.

53. Sheldon, J. J., Russin, L. A., Gargano, F. P.: Lumbar spinal stenosis. Radiographic diagnosis with special reference to transverse axial tomography. *Clin. Orthop. 115:*53–67, 1976.

54. Epstein, J. A., Epstein, B. S., Lavine, L. S., Carras, R., Rosenthal, A. D., Sumnar, P.: Lumbar nerve root compression at the intervertebral foramina caused by arthritis of the posterior facets. *J. Neurosurg. 39:*362–369, 1973.

55. Ehni, G.: Significance of the small lumbar spinal canal: cauda equina compression syndromes due to spondylosis. Parts 1–4. *J. Neurosurg. 31:*490–512, 1969.

56. Verbiest, H.: A radicular syndrome from developmental narrowing of the lumbar vertebral canal. *J. Bone Joint Surg. 36B:*236, 1954.

57. Verbiest, H.: Further experiences on the pathological influence of a developmental narrowness of the lumbar vertebral canal. *J. Bone Joint Surg. 37B:*576, 1955.

58. Newman, P. H.: Stenosis of the lumbar spine in spondylolisthesis. *Clin. Orthop. 115:*116, 1976.

59. Cauchoix, J., Benoist, M., Chassaing, V.: Degenerative spondylolisthesis. *Clin. Orthop. 115:*122, 1976.

60. Epstein, J. A., Epstein, B. S., Lavine, L. S., Carras, R., Rosenthal, A. D.: Degenerative lumbar spondylolisthesis with an intact neural arch (pseudo spondylolisthesis). *J. Neurosurg. 44:*139–147, 1976.

61. Colley, C. P., Dunsker, S. B.: Traumatic narrowing of the dorsolumbar spinal canal demonstrated by computed tomography. *Radiology 120:*95–98, 1978.

62. Kane, W.: Incidence of Laminectomy in U.S.A., Seventh Annual Meeting of the International Society for the study of the Lumbar Spine, New Orleans, LA, May 26, 1980.

63. Burton, C. V., Nida, G.: Be good to your back, Sister Kenny Institute, Minneapolis, MN, Publication 738, 1980.

64. Crock, H. V.: Observations on the management of failed spinal operations. *J. Bone Joint Surg. 58-B:*193–199, 1976.

65. Finneson, B. E.: A lumbar disc surgery predictive score card. *Spine 3:*186–188, 1978.

66. Quencer, R. M., Murtagh, F. R., Post, M. J., Rosomoff, H. L., Stokes, N. A.: Postoperative bony stenosis of the lumbar spinal canal: Evaluation of 164 symptomatic patients with axial radiography. *A.J.R. 131:*1059–1064, 1978.

67. Wiltse, L. L.: Quoted in the Medical News section. *J.A.M.A. 229:*376, 1974.

68. Gill, G. G., Sakovich, L., Thompson, E.: Pedicle fat grafts for the prevention of scar formation after laminectomy. *Spine 4:*176–186, 1978.

69. Brodsky, A. E.: Post-laminectomy and post-fusion stenosis of the lumbar spine. *Clin. Orthop. 115:*130–139, 1976.

70. Shenkin, H. A., Hash, C. J.: A new approach to the surgical treatment of lumbar spondylosis. *J. Neurosurg. 44:*148–155, 1976.

71. Wiltse, L. L., Kirkaldy-Willis, W. H., and McIvor, G. W. D.: The treatment of spinal stenosis. *Clin. Orthop. 115:*83, 1976.

72. Mooney, V.: Symposium: Spine Fusion. Seventh Annual Meeting of the International Society for study of the Lumbar Spine. New Orleans, LA, May 27, 1980.

4

Patient Selection for Lumbar Disc Surgery

All of us who practice surgery wish to exercise good surgical judgment. With lumbar disc surgery, the most critical factors involved in proper judgment relate to the indications for bringing the patient into the operating room. Decision-making regarding patient selection varies considerably from surgeon to surgeon. Being in a position to see many patients who have not fared well after lumbar disc surgery, I wish to acknowledge a personal bias, that all too often, disc surgeons seek surgical solutions to what may not necessarily be surgical problems.

This section is submitted to put forward three separate but inter-related postulates:

(1) The single most important factor relating to outcome of lumbar disc surgery is proper patient selection.

(2) Criteria for surgery based on pain, that most subjective and difficult to assess symptom, may have as many variables as there are individual surgeons. The use of a scoring system in which numerical values are assigned to the various criteria may allow us to communicate more easily about this complex problem.

(3) The passage of years is associated with structural and mechanical changes in the lumbar spine introducing a temporal factor. Improvement of old symptoms from the originally involved interspace and development of new symptoms from a previously asymptomatic interspace may occur. This temporal factor makes long-term patient selection assessment multidimensional.

The data for this association of ideas is based on two papers originally presented in the form of preliminary reports to "The International Society for the Study of the Lumbar Spine" in 1977 and 1978, and subsequently published in *Spine* in 1978 and 1979.[1, 2]

"LOW BACK LOSERS"

In the past decade, much attention has been given to the increasing problem of the unimproved patient after lumbar disc surgery. Because of persisting symptoms after surgery, additional lumbar spinal surgery may be performed under the banner of "we must do something for this poor suffering patient." All too often, well-intentioned surgeons who carry out repeat lumbar spine surgery are bludgeoned into the realization that no matter how severe or how intractable the pain, it can always be made worse by surgery. Because the failed low-back syndrome is generally associated with a normal life span, the reservoir of such patients is progressively cumulative.

Every year, we see approximately 200 patients at the Crozer-Chester Medical Center Low Back Pain Clinic who have had unsuccessful lumbar spine surgery. Some of these people are badly crippled, both physically and emotionally. Since they have fared poorly in the hands of the medical establishment, they often relate to physicians with hostility, fear, and distrust. A glum despondency often is seen in these individuals who have reached a discouraging state of chronic invalidism. Excessive use of and dependency upon narcotics and medication is common. In some instances, their lives are ruined. In those situations, I sometimes think it may be worse than cancer, since we can at least look forward to death solving the problem. These people will not die from their lumbar spine problems.

WHAT CAUSES A POOR SURGICAL RESULT?

Ninety-four patients with failed low-back syndromes were referred for consultation to the Crozer-Chester Medical Center Low Back Pain Clinic during the period from July to December, 1976. A detailed history was taken and a physical examination was performed on each patient. Some patients were accompanied by complete past medical records and roentgenogram studies; others had incomplete records and roentgenogram studies. All such data were carefully reviewed when available. A total of 179 lumbar spine operative procedures have been performed on these patients by 46 surgeons (Table 4.1).

Careful review of this relatively small series was carried out in an effort to determine if some common factors could be identified which might be of etiologic significance in the production of the failed low-back syndrome. A critical assessment of this material demonstrated that the single most striking factor influencing the outcome of surgery is poor patient selection before the initial operative procedure.

As is true with any retrospective study, the benefit of hindsight may create a bias, particularly when attempting to assess a skill as subjective as clinical judgment. With this caveat in mind, the author nevertheless holds to his opinion that the original surgery was not indicated in 76 of the 94 (81%) cases reviewed.

IMPORTANCE OF PATIENT SELECTION

If the primary cause of the poor surgical result in the low back patient is inadequate presurgical patient selection, it seems timely to stimulate discussion regarding this issue. It is necessary for the spine surgeon to be able to recognize who is likely to benefit from surgery and, possibly even more important for him, to identify the patient who is apt to do poorly after surgery. The most that we can reasonably expect, even if the finest surgeon operates on a patient who does not need surgery, is the creation of only minimal iatrogenic dysfunction superimposed on the original problem. Under less optimal circumstances, limitless complications may result.

FORMULATION OF SCORE CARD

The predictive score card (Table 4.2) is conceived of not as a finished product but more in terms of a preliminary report which may stimulate dialogue leading to generally accepted criteria for lumbar disc surgery.

All medical judgments, relating to therapy, are made by assigning positive and negative relative values to various aspects of the clinical picture, with the final decision made by balancing out these relative values. A numerical value system is not commonly used, but such a system may allow us to communicate more easily about this complex problem. The only absolute indication for lumbar disc surgery is the cauda equina syndrome, which is a surgical emergency. All other indications are relative, with the chief indication being pain. Any surgical judgment that is based pri-

Table 4.1. Frequency of surgery in 94 patients studied

Patients (no.)	Operative procedures (no.)
41	1
33	2
12	3
5	4
2	5
1	6

Table 4.2. Lumbar disc surgery predictive score card

This questionnaire is of predictive value when limited to candidates for excision of a herniated lumbar disc who have not previously undergone lumbar spine surgery. It is not designed to encompass candidates for other types of lumbar spine surgery such as decompressive laminectomy or fusion.

Positive points	Positive factors	Negative factors	Negative points
5	1. Low back and sciatic pain severe enough to be incapacitating	1. Back pain primarily	15
15	2. Sciatica is more severe than back pain	2. Gross obesity	10
5	3. Weight bearing (sitting or standing) aggravates the pain; bed rest (in some position) eases the pain	3. Nonorganic signs and symptoms—entire leg numb; simultaneous weakness of flexion and tension of toes; extension of pain into areas not explainable by organic lesion	10
25	4. Neurologic examination demonstrates a single root syndrome indicating a specific interspace	4. Poor psychologic background—attempted suicide, unrealistically high expectations from surgery; previous admissions for nonorganic symptoms—hyperventilation—unexplainable chest pains and abdominal pains—intractable incisional pain; alcoholic; not happy with job; physical demands of present occupation excessive; hostility to environment—employer—spouse; much time off from work for medical reasons (man out of work 6 months—woman out of work 16 months)	15
25	5. Myelographic defect corroborating the neurologic examination	5. Secondary gain—work connected accident; vehicular accident; medico-legal adversary situation; near retirement age—eligible for disability pension if symptoms persist	20
10	6. Positive straight leg raising test	6. History of previous law suits for medico-legal problems	10
20	Crossed straight leg raising test		
10	7. Patient's realistic self-appraisal of future life style		

Positive total ☐

Negative total ☐

Subtract negative total from positive total ☐ for predictive number

SCORING	
75 and over	Good
65–75	Fair
55–65	Marginal
Below 55	Poor

marily on such a subjective symptom as pain can have as many variables as there are surgeons.

A review of charts of 296 patients who had undergone lumbar disc surgery was carried out. Of these, 200 patients had good results and 96 patients had poor results from lumbar disc surgery. Of the 13 factors utilized in the score card, (Table 4.2), four positive factors (3, 4, 5, and 6) and two negative factors (2 and 5), or a total of six factors, were readily retrieved from old records; three positive factors (1, 2, and 7) and four negative factors (1, 3, 4, and 6) or a total of seven factors could not be readily retrieved from the old records and were derived from detailed interviews of the 96 patients with failed back syndromes.

POSITIVE SCORE CARD FACTORS

Factor 1. The key word is "incapacitating." If pain is not severe enough to hamper activities of daily living, the patient often will be dissatisfied with the results of surgery.

Factor 2. Excision of a herniated lumbar disc usually will relieve nerve root pain. If sciatica is not the major symptom and surgery provides relief of sciatica but no improvement of the back pain, the unhappy patient may well ignore the disappearance of the minor sciatica and concentrate on the persisting predominant back pain.

Factor 3. Body position should affect a lumbar disc syndrome if it is indeed a mechanical problem. Sciatic syndromes that are unaffected by changes in body position are often nonmechanical in nature and will not be alleviated by mechanical removal of pressure.

Factor 4. Self-explanatory (see Table 4.2).

Factor 5. It is important that the myelographic defect corroborates the neurologic examination. We must keep in mind the various reports that indicate percentages varying from 25–35% of abnormal lumbar myelograms in (low-back) syndrome-free patients.

Factor 6. The straight leg raising test is a good predictive factor. The crossed leg raising test (the nonpainful leg is raised which produces aggravation of pain radiating into the painful leg) is twice as effective.

Factor 7. This is an important factor that may easily be ignored by the surgeon. The only way to appreciate the patient's postoperative expectations is to spend some time listening to the patient.

NEGATIVE SCORE CARD FACTORS

Factor 1. This is the reverse of positive Factor 2.

Factor 2. Although initially, grossly obese people seem to do about the same as those with a more normal habitus, after 1 or 2 years, the recurrence rate is somewhat higher.

Factor 3. Simultaneous weakness of great toe flexion and extension cannot be explained by pressure on a single root and, unless some neurologic explanation can be offered for this finding, it should be considered nonorganic.

Factor 4. This is a "mixed bag," but any of these factors should cause the surgeon to be cautious. The alcoholic, for example, may have demonstrated a very steady work history in the past and never may have been hospitalized previously. It should be recognized, however, that these people arise every morning and set about their tasks only with great effort and difficulty. Any break in their routine may produce a behavior reversal.

Factors 5 and 6. Self-explanatory (see Table 4.2).

ELECTROMYOGRAPHY

Electromyographic (EMG) testing may be useful in several situations. If a patient manifests a sciatic syndrome of equivocal organicity, a normal EMG will be helpful. It is not used as a criterion influencing the decision to operate. If surgery is decided upon, I will not use the EMG to help me decide at which level to operate.

CAT SCAN OF LUMBAR SPINE

This most valuable x-ray technique provides important information that neither the plain lumbar spine films nor the myelogram can provide—an adequate demonstration of the configuration and size of the spinal canal. Such information is most helpful in determining what type of surgery is most suitable. For example, when a capacious spinal canal is demonstrated, a simple disc excision may be adequate, but the same myelographic defect in a stenotic canal may require a decompressive laminectomy. Recent innovations allowing visualization of disc protrusion may eventually eliminate the need for routine myelography.

RETROSPECTIVE EVALUATION

As a logical second step to determine the validity of the predictive number, a retrospective score card analysis of patients who previously had undergone lumbar disc surgery was undertaken.

The charts of 596 patients who had undergone lumbar disc surgery at the Crozer-Chester Medical Center between the years 1962–1974 were reviewed and each patient was scored using the lumbar disc surgery predictive score card. After the predictive number had been assigned, mailings were sent to each of the 596 patients. The mailing included a form letter requesting self-evaluation of the results of their lumbar disc surgery and a self-addressed postcard on which were printed four blocks labeled 1–4 (Fig. 4.1).

For purposes of adapting the patients' mailed self-assessment to the score card, the responses were graded as follows: 1, good; 2, fair; 3, marginal; and 4, poor.

From the 596 mailings, there were 303 responses, 23 of which were not considered suitable for inclusion in the study. Several responses which were considered unsuita-

Dear (*patient's name*):

I am writing to obtain your assessment of the lumbar disc surgery I performed on (*date*).

To facilitate your response, I have enclosed a self-addressed postcard. Please check the number (on the postcard) which most closely describes your present condition.

1. If, after surgery, your pain was improved and you were able to function well, please check #1.
2. If your pain was improved but you were not able to function without occasional medication and occasional time off from your activities, please check #2.
3. If, after surgery, your pain was improved but you still have considerable discomfort that requires frequent medication and time off from your activities, please check #3.
4. If, after surgery, you are either unimproved or worse, please check #4.

I have provided a space on the postcard (COMMENTS) for any additional information you may wish to include.

Thank you in advance for your help.

Bernard E. Finneson, M.D.

Figure 4.1.

ble were those in which the patient had died and a numerical assessment was submitted by the spouse. The rest were patients who did not understand the instructions and checked more than one block. One hundred forty-three mailings (24%) were returned marked "addressee unknown." Four hundred forty-six (75%) were accounted for. No answer was received nor was the envelope returned marked addressee unknown from 150 (25%).

RESULTS

The 280 patients submitting suitable responses indicated self-assessment of their lumbar disc surgery as shown in Table 4.3.

The time interval between surgery and score card evaluation of the 280 patients varied from 3–16 years with a mean follow-up duration of 8.4 years.

The predictive numbers of each result category were averaged and are shown in Table 4.4.

A comparison of the average predictive number with the scoring box at the bottom of the score card is shown in Table 4.5.

The average predictive numbers of the good and fair categories fall within the suggested parameters but the marginal and poor categories demonstrate no significant difference. Further, it is apparent that the numerical differences between the various categories are not great. The average predictive number for the good category is just above the permissible score of 75. The fair, marginal, and poor categories numerically are so close to each other that one would hesitate to accept these figures as being statistically meaningful.

ASSESSMENT OF SHORT-TERM RESULTS

Since the score card appeared to be of meager benefit in assessing the long-term follow-up patient, we analyzed the 83 patients (of the basic 280 patient sampling) who had undergone surgery in 1973, 1974,

and 1975 with a mean follow-up duration of 3.8 years (Table 4.6).

The predictive numbers of each result category were averaged and are shown in Table 4.7.

A comparison of the average predictive number with the scoring box at the bottom of the score card is shown in Table 4.8.

In comparison to the basic 280 patient sampling, the average predictive numbers of the 83 patients with a mean follow-up duration of 3.8 years fall more clearly within the anticipated parameters of the score

Table 4.3. Patients' self-assessment responses

Result	Number	Percent
Good	222	79.3
Fair	22	7.8
Marginal	25	8.9
Poor	11	4.0
Total	280	100

Table 4.4 Predictive numbers for each category

Result	Average predictive number
Good	75.8
Fair	66.3
Marginal	62.9
Poor	62.3

Table 4.5. Comparison of average predictive number and scoring box

Scoring	Result	Average predictive number
>75	Good	75.8
65–75	Fair	66.3
55–65	Marginal	62.9
<55	Poor	62.3

Table 4.6. Analysis of 83 patients

Result	Number	Percent
Good	64	77.2
Fair	10	12.0
Marginal	7	8.4
Poor	2	2.4
Total	83	100

Table 4.7. Predictive numbers of each category

Result category	Predictive number
Good	78.1
Fair	67.7
Marginal	62
Poor	55

Table 4.8. Comparison of average predictive number with scoring box

Scoring	Result	Average predictive number
>75	Good	78.1
65–75	Fair	67.7
55–65	Marginal	62
<55	Poor	55

card. The numerical differences between the various categories are reasonably disparate and probably can be classified as statistically significant.

ANSWERS TO QUESTIONS THAT WERE NOT ASKED

This investigative effort provides answers to questions that were not asked.

The reason that the selection criteria were not especially relevant in the long-term follow-up patient lies in the progressively evolving nature of the lumbar discs. The damaged disc that goes on to herniate leads to hypertrophic osteoarthritic changes that may eventually yield a relatively nonmobile painless joint. Such a self-created fusion may place increased stress on the originally painless adjacent interspace and, in time, cause a totally new set of symptoms. So, as a result of this ever-changing, adapting, magic structure called the lumbar spine, the individual who underwent lumbar disc surgery 16 years ago is not the same patient who mailed in a response to my form letter.

This dynamic mechanical evolution causes me to avoid the word "cure" in discussing low back dysfunction. I have been actively involved in the treatment of low back dysfunction since 1950; and do not claim to have ever cured anyone, although I like to think that I have benefited my fair share.

References

1. Finneson, B. E.: A lumbar disc surgery predictive score cord. *Spine* 3(2):June 1978.
2. Finneson, B. E., Cooper, V. R.: A lumbar disc surgery predictive score card: A retrospective evaluation. *Spine* 4(2):March/April 1979.

5

Microlumbar Discectomy: A Surgical Alternative for Initial Disc Herniation

INTRODUCTION

The surgical microscope with its high-intensity light source and recording accessories becomes a fascinating tool for many surgeons. As a visual aid for traditional surgical procedures, operating time and blood loss are noticeably reduced as surgical techniques become progressively more accurate. Although the instrument requires consistent use for proficiency, its limitations seem only those of manual dexterity and imagination.

For spine surgeons interested in the potentials of magnification, the lumbar anatomy proved a readily available laboratory model for microsurgical experience. The structure most afflicted by clinical disease was, of course, the intervertebral disc. Reduction in wound size with strict adherence to avascular tissue planes made possible by the concentrated light source and magnification resulted in meticulous hemostasis necessary for clarity of the microsurgical field. Apparent clinical rewards were a remarkable reduction in surgical morbidity and convalescence.

Such has been the fascination of this author for the potentials of microsurgery in the treatment of benign lumbar nerve root compression syndromes. The availability of the operating microscope encourages re-evaluation of accepted surgical principles and techniques. Initial reports were presented on the postsurgical tissue morbidity of patients with failed disc syndrome.[1, 2] Eventually, this experience provided the stimulus for development of microlumbar discectomy, a totally microsurgical operative technique introduced for the treatment of initial lumbar disc herniations.[2, 3] Emphasis was placed on a reconsideration of accepted methods for penetration of the annulus fibrosus and the volume of disc material that must necessarily be removed at first surgery to minimize spontaneous disc reherniations.[4, 5] An apparent relationship surfaced between the preservation of extradural fat and delayed adhesion reactions, while a means was suggested to modify surgical wounds in the annulus fibrosus that might preserve better its competence to withstand subsequent intervertebral stress.[5] Instrumentation was introduced in 1977, allowing the potential benefits of a microsurgical approach to the herniated lumbar disc to be more widely evaluated.[3, 5, 6] The summary of opinions by all authors on the subject indicates a marked reduction in surgical morbidity is possible when the operating microscope is utilized for a more accurate and less traumatic approach to the lumbar intervertebral space.[6, 7]

OBSERVATIONS ON TISSUE MORBIDITY AFTER FAILED LUMBAR SURGERY

Since April 1972, the author has utilized the surgical microscope in the treatment of 754 cases of initial lumbar disc herniations. An additional 226 patients with failed lumbar surgeries have also been operated. This latter group represents 95 re-explorations after initial microlumbar discectomy and 131 patients whose first surgical procedure was titled either lumbar laminectomy or lumbar laminectomy with spinal fusion. Microsurgical observations on normal and postsurgical lumbar tissue deserve special comment.

Individual Tissue Morbidity

Skin and Skin Incisions

Large mid-line and transverse skin incisions frequently are hyperesthetic and painful to touch. This is true especially of scars over the iliac crest in spinal fusion patients. When present, palpable nodules acting as trigger zones have been removed and histologic study suggests neuromas. Painful cutaneous scars have not been observed when midline longitudinal microsurgical incisions are used to approach the lumbar anatomy.

Subcutaneous Tissue

This layer may atrophy after surgical disturbance. When the subcutaneous tissue shrinks, nonabsorbable suture material often becomes palpable and dysesthetic to touch. Such postsurgical reactions are unpredictable, occurring more commonly in females. This observation suggests that suture material of minimal diameter tied with inverted knots might provide the most silent wound closure. Microsurgical incisions seldom require repair of the subcutaneous layer.

Paravertebral Fascia

The lumbar fascia scars minimally when a midline incision is used. Paramedian and transverse openings, however, frequently heal with muscle herniations through the fascia. Since muscle seems well-supplied with somatic pain fibers, a correlation between chronic postsurgical muscle spasm and fascial incisions other than midline is not surprising.

Large wounds approximated with fascial sutures of nonabsorbable material are frequently painful to pressure. This problem seems avoided, however, if midline microsurgical incisions are used.

Paravertebral Muscle

The paralumbar muscles should be treated gently during surgical dissections. When traumatized, muscle will bleed considerably and hemostasis may prove difficult without the use of electrocautery. The end result will be dense muscle scars from electrical burns. Microsurgical incisions will greatly reduce any need for muscle retraction and hemostasis.

The transverse fixation of longitudinal muscle masses across the midline with suture material is common practice in large wound closures. Such a practice well may contribute to the postsurgical kinetic pain frequently experienced by these patients.

Ligamentum Flavum

This ligament is attached densely to the periosteum of the lamina and fans laterally into the depths of the spinal recesses. The structure varies greatly in mass and distribution and, at times, appears paper-thin, affording little protection in the deeper neural tissue during surgical approach to the intervertebral disc. Penetration of the ligamentum flavum requires extreme caution, as rupture into the subarachnoid space may otherwise occur.

The normal ligament serves to separate the deeper neural structures from overlying muscle and bone. Once removed, however, it does not regenerate. When considerable ligamentum flavum has been removed at first surgery, a thick fibrous scar often results, filling the interlaminar space and growing downward into the extradural canal. Dense adhesions to the underlying nerve root can be expected. Lysis of such attachments are often difficult and easily complicated by unrecognized dural tears. If the arachnoid remains intact, pulsatile cystic herniations of this structure through a dural laceration may result, reaching considerable size and further compressing the neural structures. In addition, full thickness microscopic tears in the meninges, invisible to the naked eye, frequently have proved the source of recurring "seromas" in postlaminectomy patients.

A major sacrifice of ligamentum flavum at first surgery predicts dense adhesions as the etiology of postsurgical sciatic pain. Such patients may respond dramatically to tedious microsurgical dissection, but an insidious return of their radiculitis will not be surprising. Postsurgical adhesion sciatica has been rare after microlumbar discectomy where maximal preservation of the ligamentum flavum is stressed at initial surgery.[3, 5, 7]

The Lamina

Microsurgical re-exploration of patients treated initially with laminectomy and fusion procedures often reveals considerable change in the lamina. When rongeurs are used, regenerative osteoblastic activity may occur with extreme focal thickening of the lamina and downward growth of osteophytes. As a result, the associated lateral recess is often wedged, trapping the nerve root. The condition is suspected when smooth postsurgical myelographic defects are seen and often can be predicted by computed tomographic (CT) scanning which demonstrates unilateral bony distortions of the neural canal. Additionally, hypertrophy of the ligamentum flavum is often observed with partial laminectomy and may contribute considerably to the mass effect of regenerative osteophytes against an already compromised nerve root. These findings suggest that central laminectomy sparing the facets and lateral recesses will

incur less morbidity than lateral rongeuring of the lamina, assuming that the ligamentum flavum remains to protect the neural elements from postsurgical adhesions.

The Facet

The lumbar facets minimize vertebral rotatory movements and prevent subluxation. The joint and its synovium are richly supplied with somatic innervation, as demonstrated by facet pain syndrome. Denervation of the joint by anesthetic injection and stereotactic procedures has often been recommended for this condition.

Microsurgical study of postsurgical patients with facet pain has been rewarding. In the normal state, the joint surface lies obliquely vertical and is invisible. If the most lateral fibers of the ligamentum flavum are removed, however, the synovial membrane of the facet will often balloon into the surgical defect. It can be recognized easily as a white, glistening inflated pouch.

In postlaminectomy patients with facet pain, however, the bony plates will prove to be rongeured and the synovial balloon destroyed. Osteoblastic distortions of the joint and withered hyperemic residuals of the synovium are all that remain. Postsurgical facet pain has been unresponsive to reoperation and microsurgical observations in these patients suggest the surgical rongeur as a major etiologic factor.

Lateral Bony Spinal Canal and Foramen

The lateral spinal canal presents as a smooth bony surface in the patient without degenerative disc disease. When rongeurs are applied for surgical exposure, the mouth of the instrument can produce sharp bony spicules approximating each bite. Such projections are visible with magnification and often appear to spur the approximating nerve root on its lateral surface.

After foraminotomy, a napkin-ring type constriction of the nerve root by soft bone resembling osteophyte frequently has been observed at the foramen entrance. Whether this is the direct result of regenerative attempts within the foramen after instrumentation or a natural process of aging remains unclear. Reviewing initial operative reports in an attempt to correlate cause and effect of this phenomenon has proved unrewarding. It can be said, however, that the word "foraminotomy" covers a myriad of surgical alterations to the neural window. Since the foramen lies hidden from vertical view unless wide decompressions are used, the structure would seem best avoided for fear of generating an iatrogenic etiology for postsurgical sciatic pain.

Extradural Fat

Fat tissue in the normal spinal canal is abundant, lobulated, and well vascularized. Although easily retracted and preserved with micro-operative techniques,[3, 5] the tissue often seems sacrificed for better exposure during laminectomy operations. Microsurgical study of such patients with recurrent sciatica reveals extremely dense adhesion reactions in the neural canal. Perhaps the tissue was not really sacrificed, but simply atrophied after surgical manipulation. This seems unlikely, however, as disappearance of fat has not been observed after microsurgical techniques where the tissue is protected. Whatever the mechanism involved, the presence of extradural fat in the postoperative spinal canal seems critical for preservation of anatomical planes.[5, 8, 9] Without it, a dense fibrous postsurgical adhesion reaction can be expected.

Extradural Veins

Abundant and dilated venous structures in the spinal canal are characteristic of degenerative disc disease.[8] Under magnification, the engorgement of these vessels disappears dramatically with decompression of the disc hernia. In patients with tight bony canals and small disc hernias, it is reasonable to speculate that markedly distended veins may add significantly to nerve root compression.

In reviewing operative reports of patients with postsurgical sciatica who received transfusions at initial surgery, electrocautery has surfaced as the technique of choice for hemostasis. At microsurgical re-exploration, severe granulation masses were observed to fill the extradural space, with dense, fibrous scars appearing on the dura and nerve roots. These lesions surely represent the healing of electrical burns, a surgical morbidity for which there is no treatment. The use of magnification at initial disc surgery virtually will eliminate hemorrhage and the need for transfusions.[5]

Posterior Longitudinal Ligament

This ligament reinforces the annulus fibrosus of the disc in the midline. Undoubtedly, this explains the high incidence of lateral disc herniations. The normal structure is glistening, white, and avascular. With aging or surgical insult, however, the ligament turns grayish and often separates widely from the annulus. This fact proves important as a pocket may be formed which conceals significant amounts of extruded disc material. When a clinical picture of undulating postoperative sciatica appears after initial intervertebral decompression, a mass of disc material packed between the annulus fibrosus and posterior longitudinal ligament should be suspected. It is difficult to view this area of anatomy even with magnification. Knowledge of its existence, however, will allow the surgeon to gently explore for such extrusions, thus minimizing the possibility of postsurgical undulating disc syndrome.[5]

Annulus Fibrosus and Intervertebral Disc

The annulus fibrosus is a multilayered avascular retaining wall for the nucleus pulposus of the disc. When the structure becomes incompetent to intervertebral pressures, the disc will rupture. It seems that degenerative disc disease is really a disease of annulus fibrosus.[5]

It is common practice to open the annulus by scalpel incision. It can be demonstrated easily at reoperation, however, that the annulus fibrosus heals poorly and only by fibrous secondary intention once surgically lacerated.[5] As true recurrent disc herniations rarely have been recorded by this author without a gaping wound in the annulus fibrosus, a technique of dilating the annulus, rather than scalpel incision, is suggested for best preservation of function.[3, 5]

The histology of disc material changes dramatically once curetted. Healthy resilient fibroelastic tissue soon will become edematous and friable. If the purpose of curettement is to allow for maximal disc decompression and prevention of spontaneous reherniations, the spine surgeon should measure his proficiency with this maneuver in the autopsy room. Utilizing all standard and microsurgical operative approaches available in the living patient, it has been impossible for this author to remove more than 50% of the contents of a healthy intervertebral space regardless of the instrumentation and diligence applied. Such an experience suggests that curettement severely macerates disc material that will remain after first surgery. Such a maneuver well may increase the possibility of spontaneous disc reherniations, especially when the annulus fibrosus has been lacerated by scalpel incision.

In the multioperated lumbar patient who receives repeated curettements, the intervertebral space can eventually be evacuated. Such individuals are often characterized by "kissing bone" syndrome in which lumbar pain and sciatica will rapidly recur on weight bearing, having been relieved by a prolonged period of flat bed rest.[5] The mechanism suggested is an approximation of the vacant disc space under body weight that subluxes the facet plates and mechanically narrows the foramen, thus recompressing the nerve root.

CONCLUSIONS ON POSTSURGICAL TISSUE MORBIDITY

Microsurgical evaluation of postsurgical lumbar tissue shows dramatic changes in gross histology. The paraspinal muscles will be densely scarred by surgical incisions off the midline, especially when electrocautery instruments are used for hemostasis. Wherever bone is disturbed by rongeuring, regenerative osteoblastic activity is often visible with osteophyte formations spurring the nerve root or trapping it by mass effect in the associated lateral recess. Anatomical planes disappear with sacrifice of ligamentum flavum and extradural fat. The annulus fibrosus does not heal by primary intention after scalpel laceration, possibly promoting further incompetence of its retaining wall to subsequent intervertebral pressures.[5] Curettement of the disc space will macerate healthy disc material, much of which will remain as a residuum even after the most vigorous evacuation attempts at first surgery. Although an evacuated space can eventually be achieved by multiple curettements, a syndrome of weight-bearing sciatica will frequently result. Finally, the density and mass of postsurgical adhesions seems directly related to the disappearance of extradural fat and the use of electrocautery techniques for hemostasis in the spinal canal.

DESIGNING A MICROSURGICAL TECHNIQUE FOR INITIAL LUMBAR DISC HERNIATIONS

Based upon observations of tissue morbidity gained through microsurgical re-exploration of patients with failed lumbar surgeries, certain technical principles seem critical if maximal success is to be achieved in the surgical treatment of initial lumbar disc herniations. The surgeon should:

(1) minimize soft tissue trauma by the use of small accurately placed midline skin incisions.
(2) avoid electrocoagulation and suture approximation of muscle.
(3) allow no rongeuring of the lamina or facet.
(4) preserve a maximal amount of ligamentum flavum.

(5) preserve extradural fat.

(6) visualize and protect the nerve root at all times.

(7) dilate an opening in the annulus fibrosus, rather than using scalpel incisions.

(8) avoid currettage of the disc space or remove excessive amounts of healthy disc material.

(9) achieve hemostasis in the extradural canal without electrocautery techniques.

(10) minimize foreign materials during wound closure.

The operating microscope provides the means to decompress a herniated lumbar disc while respecting these surgical principles. An operative procedure designed for this purpose has been titled microlumbar discectomy (MLD).[3, 5]

MICROLUMBAR DISCECTOMY

Surgical Microscope

A Zeiss OPMI #1 surgical microscope with 400-mm lens is used to perform this operation. The patient is placed in the prone position and the surgeon stands on the same side as the herniated disc undergoing treatment. The microscope stand and scrub nurse are stationed opposite the surgeon. The surgical microscope is used during the entire operative procedure from skin incision to skin closure.

Surgical Instruments (Fig. 5.1)

The surgical instruments used for the procedure are the Williams' microlumbar discectomy retractors, disc forceps, and suction retractor (Fig. 5.1).*

Anesthesia and Positioning (Fig. 5.2)

General endotracheal anesthesia assisted by a mechanical ventilator is the anesthetic technique of choice for this operation.

The patient is turned to the prone position on an Olympic VAC PAC #30† support

---

* Codman and Shurtleff, Inc., Randolph, MA.
† Olympic Medical Corp., Seattle, WA.

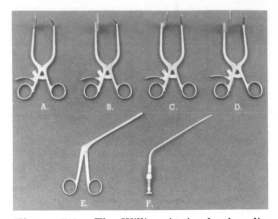

Figure 5.1. The Williams' microlumbar discectomy instruments are pictured, consisting of self-retaining retractors, disc forceps, and nerve root suction retractor.

with an inflated bladder lying directly under the abdomen (Fig. 5.2). The VAC PAC is then moulded tightly under the patient during inspiration and hardened by suction. When the bladder is deflated, a vacant space is created under the abdomen which reduces intraspinal pressure and extradural venous engorgement. In addition, respiratory movements which can disturb the depth of field during the use of high magnification are minimized by this technique.

Skin Incision (Fig. 5.3)

A midline 1-inch skin incision when accurately placed is sufficient to expose and decompress a herniated lumbar disc. Larger incisions increase surgical morbidity and hinder the meticulous hemostasis that is crucial for clarity of the microsurgical field.

The anatomical relationship of a palpable spinous process to its deeper lamina varies greatly from L3 to S1. A direct vertical approach to the lower three interlaminar spaces is best obtained if the skin incisions are marked according to Figure 5.3. At the L3–L4 level, the incision should be directly over the L3 spinous process. An L4–L5 approach requires an incision over the lower portion of the L4 spine and extends slightly downward over the interspinous space. At L5–S1, the incision is made directly over

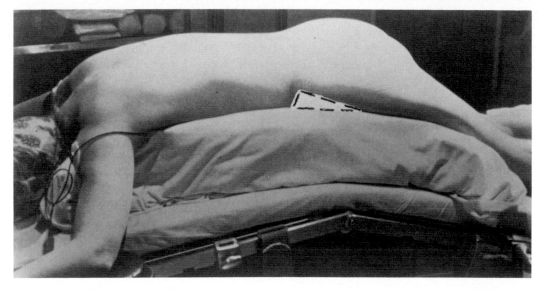

Figure 5.2.   The prone position is used during microlumbar discectomy. A vacant space is present under the abdomen which allows the abdomen to sag with respirations, thus reducing intraspinal pressures and venous engorgement.

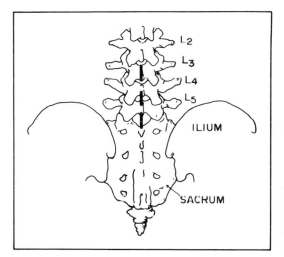

Figure 5.3.   Skin incisions for microsurgical approach to the lower lumbar intervertebral spaces should be placed as shown in this diagram. Larger incisions only contribute to difficulties in hemostasis and postsurgical morbidity.

the interspinous space. When it is difficult to localize the level for exploration by palpation of surface anatomy alone, a lateral lumbar radiogram is taken for confirmation.

Using the surgical microscope at lower magnifications, the skin is incised with a

#10 scalpel. Meticulous hemostasis is obtained in the superficial layers with bipolar coagulation. The wound must be kept dry from onset, otherwise clarity of the microsurgical field will be greatly disturbed as the dissection progresses.

Exposure to the Interlaminar Space

Fascia Incision

The paravertebral fascia is incised at its midline attachment to the appropriate spinous processes. When the opening is placed laterally, muscle bleeding will occur and hemostasis becomes difficult.

Dissection to the Lamina

A periosteal elevator is inserted into the fascia opening and directed toward the midline. Gentle lateral movements are used to separate the paravertebral muscle from the spinous processes and lamina. Bleeding points on the muscle wall are located with magnification and treated by bipolar coagulation. The index finger then is inserted through the fascia opening and the interlamina space is palpated. If uncertain as to the level of exposure, a lateral radiogram again is used for localization. The microsurgical wound retractor is now inserted with the blade lateral toward the surgeon. Excellent visualization of the interlaminar space is obtained through the 1-inch skin incision when the retractor is properly positioned.

Surgical Approach through the Ligamentum Flavum

With the paravertebral muscles retracted laterally, the ligamentum flavum and lamina are identified (Fig. 5.4). The facet will lie lateral toward the surgeon and care must be taken not to traumatize this structure or its synovial membrane. No portion of the lamina should be removed during this operative procedure.

A superficial incision is made in the ligamentum flavum with a #15 scalpel under high magnification. A Penfield #4 Dissector is used for final penetration of the deep fibers of the ligament (Fig. 5.5). This blunt instrument should not injure the nerve root

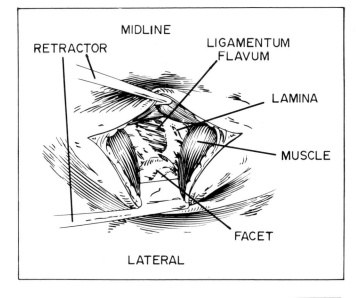

Figure 5.4. With the self-retaining retractor in place, the ligamentum flavum and surrounding lamina can be identified. The facet and its synovium lie lateral and should be protected from surgical insult.

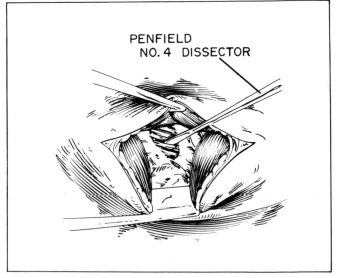

Figure 5.5. Penetration through the ligamentum flavum is made with a Penfield #4 Dissector. Care is taken not to rupture into the subarachnoid space during this maneuver.

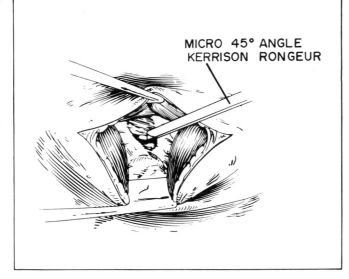

MICRO 45° ANGLE
KERRISON RONGEUR

Figure 5.6. The most lateral fibers of the ligamentum flavum are removed with a 1-mm microrongeur. The synovial membrane of the facet will often bulge into the surgical defect from its lateral position during this maneuver. Care is taken not to rupture this structure which can be identified as a glistening inflated white pouch.

or dural sac even if these structures are pressed tightly upward against the undersurface of the ligament by a large herniated disc. A 45° 1-mm rongeur is used to remove the most lateral fibers of the ligamentum flavum toward the surgeon (Fig. 5.6). The facet with its synovial membrane, bony lamina, and all extradural fat should remain intact. Meticulous hemostasis in the superfacial portion of the wound will prove critical to the ease of further dissection.

Exploration of the Extradural Space

With the lateral fibers of the ligamentum flavum removed under high magnification, a blunt 90° microhook is used to explore the extradural space. Certain features of the microsurgical anatomy in this area as they relate to herniated disc disease seem noteworthy.

The Nerve Root

Care must be taken to locate accurately and protect the nerve root during initial extradural exploration. This structure will appear white and tubular with vascular markings visible on its surface. It may lie either medial or lateral to the disc herniation. Gentle manipulation with a blunt microhook will often cause a motor response which aids the surgeon in exact localization.

In large disc herniations, the nerve root often is stretched flat and pushed directly upward toward the surgeon. In this case, the structure will appear avascular and its white, glistening surface can easily be mistaken for the annulus fibrosis of the disc. Beware!

Extradural Veins

Blood loss is minimal when high magnification is used to identify extradural veins. If rupture of these vessels does occur, proceed with the dissection and do not reduce magnification. Bleeding will stop spontaneously when the herniated disc has been decompressed. Never use pressure techniques or electrocautery to obtain hemostasis in this limited extradural exposure. Severe nerve root injury could result!

Extradural Fat

Fat should not be removed to gain better visualization in the extradural space. Although its physiologic functions in this area remain speculative, experience suggests that fat is critical in maintaining normal tissue planes and minimizing adhesions in the postoperative state.[5]

Nerve Root Retraction

With the nerve root identified, the MLD suction retractor is the only instrument required in the extradural space to maintain nerve root retraction and visualization during discectomy. The instrument is inserted with its retractor tip turned medially under the nerve root and the manifold is held between the thumb and index finger of the surgeon's nondominant hand (Fig. 5.7). The nerve root and dural sac are displaced medially by wrist movements, allowing exposure of the annulus fibrosis of the herniated disc (Fig. 5.8).

Penetration of the Annulus Fibrosis

With the suction retractor properly positioned, the annulus fibrosis of the herniated disc can be visualized. Under high magnification, this structure will appear white, glistening, fibrous, and avascular. Small tears in the annulus are often visible and indicate the possibility of extruded disc fragments in the extradural space. A 90° microhook is used to explore under the

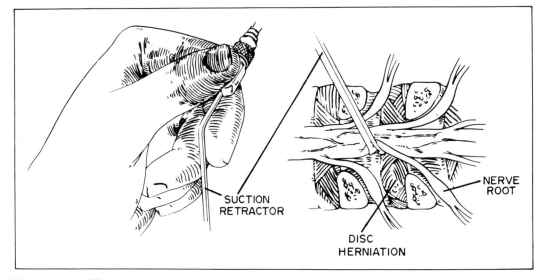

Figure 5.7.   The suction retractor is held in the surgeon's nondominant hand with the manifold between the thumb and index finger. The retractor tip is turned medial to displace the nerve root while the suction tip clears blood from the extradural space.

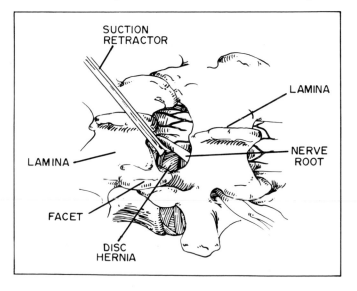

Figure 5.8.   Using gentle wrist movements, the tip of the suction retractor displaces the neural structures medially, thus exposing the annulus fibrosis of the intervertebral disc hernia.

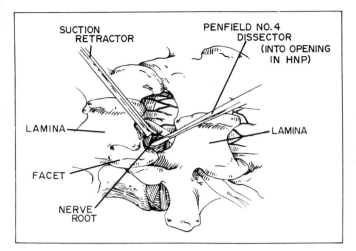

Figure 5.9. Penetration into the intervertebral disc is made by gently dilating an opening in its annulus fibrosis with a Penfield #4 dissector. This technique seems best to preserve the retaining wall function of the annulus for subsequent intervertebral stress.

neural elements mobilizing these fragments laterally when present.

In the author's experience, spontaneous recurrent disc herniations rarely occur without a gaping postsurgical wound in the annulus fibrosis. For this reason, penetration of the annulus is made with a blunt Penfield #4 Dissector (Fig. 5.9). The instrument is gently pressed through the annulus fibers and turned in a circular fashion. The result is a dilated opening which often closes in a sphincter-type fashion after decompression of the herniated disc tissue. It should be emphasized that a low incidence of recurrent disc herniations cannot be predicted with this procedure if a scalpel incision is made in the annulus fibrosis.

Decompression of the Herniated Lumbar Disc

Utilizing gentle maneuvers, the MLD forceps are pressed through the dilated opening in the annulus fibrosis. Decompression of disc tissue causing nerve root compression is accomplished by repeated small evacuations with the discectomy forceps (Fig. 5.10). The instrument has a 1-mm toothed cup and is not inserted into the disc space past the angle of the jaws. Only that volume of material which easily can be mobilized from the intervertebral space by the discectomy forceps and a 90° microhook should be removed. The disc space is

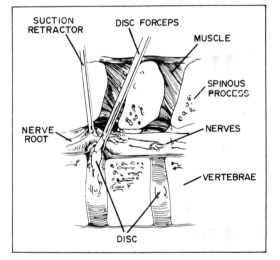

Figure 5.10. Decompression of the disc hernia is achieved by repeated small evacuations with the discectomy forceps. Curettement of the intervertebral space is not done in this surgical technique and a maximal amount of healthy disc material is allowed to remain.

not curetted in this operative procedure. When the annulus fibrosis and nerve root have been well decompressed, the suction retractor is removed. No foreign materials or solutions are placed in the extradural space prior to closure.

Wound Closure

Interrupted sutures of 3–0 nylon are used to approximate the wound. Care is taken not to suture paravertebral muscle during fascia closure. Skin sutures are removed in 10 days.

Postoperative Management

Postoperatively, the bed is kept absolutely flat although the patient may ambulate and shower as desired. Straight leg raising begins on the 2nd postoperative day (b.i.d.).

Medications postoperative include intramuscular methotrimeprazine‡ (a sedative hypnotic) and oral acetaminophen§ p.o. for pain, and oral orphenadrine‖ as a muscle relaxant. It is important to note that narcotic medications are not required for these patients during hospitalization or convalescence.

Hospital discharge occurs on the 3rd postoperative day. The patient is instructed to continue with straight leg raises indefinitely at home. Auto travel in the sitting position is restricted for 3 weeks. Swimming is encouraged after suture removal. Vocational rehabilitation for heavy manual labor and driving occupations is recommended. If indicated, a weight reduction to normal levels is stressed.

Technical Summary

The operative technique presented is designed to minimize alteration of the lumbar anatomy when surgical treatment is required for initial lumbar disc herniations. The technical principles include avoidance of laminectomy or facet trauma, preservation of all extradural fat tissue, protection of the nerve root at all times, and minimal evacuation of intervertebral disc tissue without currettement of the disc space or scalpel laceration of the annulus fibrosus.

MICROLUMBAR DISCECTOMY (MLD) SERIES

MLD, as specifically defined in this text, has been used for the treatment of 754

patients with initial lumbar disc herniations. Criteria for selection of patients include virgin lumbar anatomy (no previous lumbar surgery) and CT scan without findings of spinal stenosis. Operating time has averaged 34 minutes with a postoperative stay of 3.1 days during the past 6 years. Table 5.1 outlines the series.

Reoperation was required for a variety of conditions in 95 patients of the MLD series. One hundred and three additional surgeries have been performed in this group, bringing the total to 857 operations for the entire series of 754 patients. The reoperation series is defined as reoperative MLD series, and a record of the subsequent surgical pathology is provided in Table 5.2.

It is interesting to note that the incidence of new disc herniations (2.7 + 0.9) was 3.6%, as compared to 3.5% for true recurrent disc herniations both traumatic and spontaneous. Dilation of the annulus fibrosis and minimal discectomy appears to restore intervertebral competence at the site of initial surgery. In addition, undulating disc syndrome (1.5%) and missed discs (0.26%) have not occurred since 1977. The explanation

Table 5.1.   Microlumbar discectomy (MLD) series (April, 1972–November, 1981)

754 Patients	Initial lumbar disc herniations
Ages	18–74 years
Female	43%
Compensation cases	41%
Myelography	91%

Table 5.2.   Reoperative MLD series

	Pa- tients	% of 95	% of 754
True recurrent herniated nucleus pulposis (HNP)	27	28.4	3.5
New level HNP	20	21.1	2.7
New HNP, opposite side of 1st MLD	7	7.3	0.9
Undulating discs	11	11.6	1.5
Missed discs	2	2.1	0.3
Recurrent sciatica of postsurgical adhesions	15	15.8	2.0
Spinal stenosis	13	13.6	1.7
Total	95		

---

‡ Levoprome, Lederle Laboratories, Wayne, NJ.
§ Tylenol Extra Strength, McNeil Consumer Products, Fort Washington, PA.
‖ Norflex, Riker Laboratories, Inc., Northridge, CA.

for this is suggested to be proficiency with the MLD technique and an increasing awareness of the pitfalls of microsurgical exposure.

Thirteen patients, initially presenting as virgin disc herniations before 1978, subsequently reappeared with lumbar spinal stenosis syndromes (1.7%). Originally, all demonstrated unilateral myelographic defects and monoradiculitis. CT scanning was not available at the time of initial diagnosis, but speculation is that spinal stenosis was present but unrecognized at the time of first surgery. Initial MLD relieved root compression in all, but the onset of new lumbar and sciatic complaints prompted reinvestigation by myelography and CT scans. Congenital spinal stenosis was present in four, while the remaining nine demonstrated osteoarthritic spinal stenosis. With the exception of these 13 patients, all subsequent operations performed in the reoperative MLD series were microlumbar discectomy in type.

Recurrent sciatica from postsurgical adhesions after MLD occurred in 2.0% of the series. All of these patients had stopped straight leg raises and their initial myelographic defects were not visible on re-evaluation. MLD technique was reapplied at the original surgical site, and only gentle lysis of root adhesions were required with no further discectomy.

It should be appreciated that if patients with lumbar disc herniations and associated spinal stenosis can be accurately diagnosed and treated initially, while continuing to eliminate undulating discs and missed discs by meticulous first surgical technique, the percentage of patients subsequently entering the reoperative MLD series on a yearly basis may continue to be significantly reduced.

Finally, an analysis of reoperative treatment and its success for the 95 patients in the reoperative MLD series appears in Table 5.3. It deserves comment that all ultimate surgical failures resulted from the treatment of spontaneously occurring or

reoccuring disc protrusions. Perhaps these patients represent a true degenerative condition of the annulus fibrosis. A summary of the postoperative results for the entire MLD series appears in Table 5.4. Note carefully the definition of surgical "cure:" a patient who is economically productive if he so desires, physically comfortable without addictive medication, and free from sciatic pain.

Table 5.3. Reoperative MLD series

	Patients	Total reoperations	Failures
True recurrent HNP	27	31	1
Trauma	(17)	(17)	
Spontaneous	(10)	(14)	(√)
New level HNP	20	21	1
Trauma	(6)	(6)	
Spontaneous	(14)	(15)	(√)
New HNP, opposite side of 1st MLD	7	7	0
Trauma	(3)	(3)	
Spontaneous	(4)	(4)	
Undulating discs	11	14	4
Trauma	(1)	(2)	
Spontaneous	(10)	(12)	(√)
Missed discs	2	2	0
Recurrent sciatica of postsurgical adhesions	15	15	0
Spinal stenosis	13	13	0
Total	95	103	6

Table 5.4. Postoperative results—MLD series

Surgical "cure" is defined as a patient who is economically productive if they so desire, physically comfortable without addictive medication, and free from sciatic pain.

	Patients	% of 95	% of 754
MLD series	754		100.0
Reoperative MLD series	95(100)		12.6
Surgical cure (1st MLD)	659		87.4
Surgical cure (reoperation)	89	(93.7)	11.8
Surgical failures	6		0.8
Total 9.7-year cure after all attempts	748		99.2

CONCLUSIONS (MLD SERIES)

In this series of 754 patients with initial lumbar disc herniations, 87.4% have thus far reached surgical cure after one MLD procedure. For 95 patients in this same group who required reoperation for recurrent, continued, or entirely new lumbar sciatica syndromes, 93.7% of these ultimately reached surgical cure. The incidence of true recurrent herniated discs (same level, same side as first MLD) is 3.5%. However, 63% of these required new trauma sufficient to be treated as an emergency before decompensation occurred. Therefore, the incidence of true recurrent disc herniations after MLD, even with subsequent lumbar trauma, is not greater than the incidence of unrelated new disc herniations in this series.

There has been a satisfactory overall surgical success with this operative procedure designed specifically for initial lumbar disc herniations. Statistics suggest that the surgical technique, as defined, possibly is reconstructive in that the area of annulus fibrosis decompressed by MLD technique shows a competence equal to neighboring intervertebral areas. Surgical complications have not occurred (cerebrospinal fluid leaks or nerve root injury). Blood transfusions were required, however, in seven patients (857 operations [0.8%]). The incidence of true recurrent disc herniations which occurred spontaneously after initial MLD has been 1.3% in this 9.7-year series.

References

1. Williams, R. R. W.: The microsurgery of lumbar disc disease. American Association of Neurological Surgeons, USA, 1973.
2. Williams, R. W.: Microlumbar discectomy: a surgical technique. International College of Surgeons, USA, 1974.
3. Williams, R. W.: Microlumbar discectomy, surgical techniques. Randolph, MA, Codman and Shurtleff, Inc., 1977, p. 1.
4. Williams, R. W.: Operative results in 425 cases of herniated lumbar discs treated by microlumbar discectomy. Rocky Mountain Neurosurgical Society, USA, 1977.
5. Williams, R. W.: Microlumbar discectomy: a conservative surgical approach to the virgin herniated lumbar disc. *Spine 3(2):*175, 1978.
6. Casper, W.: A new surgical procedure for lumbar disc herniation causing less tissue damage through a microsurgical approach. In *Advances in Neurosurgery*, Vol. 4, Berlin-Heidelberg, Springer Verlag, 1977, p. 74.
7. Yasargil, M. G.: Microsurgical operation for herniated lumbar disc. In *Advances in Neurosurgery*. Vol. 4, Berlin-Heidelberg, Springer-Verlag, 1977, p. 81.
8. Williams, R. W.: Microsurgical and standard removal of the protruded lumbar disc: a comparative study: comments. *Neurosurgery 8(2):*422, 1981.
9. Wilson, D. H., Kenning, J.: Microsurgical lumbar discectomy: preliminary report of 83 consecutive cases. *Neurosurgery 4(2):*137, 1979.

Suggested Readings

1. Gilsback, J., Eggert, H. E., Seeger, W.: Microsurgery of ruptured lumbar discs. *Excerpta Medica International Congress 456:*60, 1978.
2. Gilsback, J., Eggert, H. R., Seeger, W.: Microsurgical operation for herniated lumbar disk. Aesculap, 5, Tuttlingen, Aesculap-Werke AG, 2979.
3. Goald, H. J.: Microlumbar discectomy. *Va. Med. Monthly 104:*519, 1976.
4. Goald, H. J.: Microlumbar discectomy: follow-up of 147 patients, *Spine 3(2):*183, 1978.
5. Goald, H. J.: Herniated lumbar disc treated by a new surgical procedure. In *Advances in Pain Research and Therapy*. Vol. 3, New York, NY, Raven Press, 1979, p. 719.
6. Iwa, H., Casper, W.: Microsurgery operation for lumbar disc herniation. *No Shinkei Geka 6(7):*657, 1978.
7. Williams, R. W.: Microlumbar discectomy: a surgical technique. American Association of Neurological Surgeons, USA, 1975.
8. Williams, R. W.: Microlumbar discectomy: a surgical technique with three-year follow-up (186 cases). Congress of Neurological Surgeons, USA, 1975.
9. Williams, R. W.: Microlumbar discectomy: a surgical technique with two-year follow-up. Southwest Surgical Congress, USA, 1975.
10. Williams, R. W.: Microlumbar discectomy. World Microsurgical Congress, USA, 1976.
11. Williams, R. W.: Microlumbar discectomy: operative technique and surgical results in a 5-year study (484 cases). Congress of Neurological Surgeons, USA, 1977.
12. Williams, R. W.: Microsurgical lumbar discectomy: preliminary report of 83 consecutive cases: comments. *Neurosurgery 4(2):*140, 1979.
13. Wilson, D. H., Harbaugh, R.: Microsurgical and standard removal of the protruded lumbar disc: a comparative study. *Neurosurgery 8(2):*422, 1981.

6

Neural Arch Resection

Lumbar spondylosis is a form of spinal stenosis. As a clinical entity it has been presented over the years under a variety of headings, some circumscribed and some generalized in definition. Although attempts have been made to derive a classification which includes all forms of bony encroachment, this has not been accomplished with uniform acceptance by all those who treat these problems. The reader is referred to the orthopaedic and neurosurgical literature for a review of these classifications.[1-3] Recognition of the entities, representing a collation of nonspecific clinical and radiologic findings, has not been precise until the advent of axial radiology of the lumbar spine.[4-8] For the first time, it was possible to define radiologically the types of bony abnormalities and the number of levels of involvement, a task not easily accomplished by any combination of clinical or other diagnostic techniques.

Before and even since the addition of axial radiology to the diagnostic armamentarium, the surgical response to management of bony encroachments has been varied. No single operation seemed to answer all the requirements for surgical correction of the pathologic entities seen. Perhaps this is the nature of the problem and is as it should be. However, after many years of differing surgical approaches, experiences, and reviews of the literature, a single procedure was adopted by the author which was thought to respond to the vast majority, if not all, of the bony encroachment problems. This was a procedure of neural or dorsal arch resection, based on an original technique described by Gill and associates.[9] Neural arch resection was proposed,

with removal of the entire arch at all levels of bony encroachment. The inferior and subjacent level superior articular processes were included, as suggested by any component of the clinical investigation.[10] Therefore, two elements of clinical judgment are necessary: the extent of surgical bony removal and the number of levels at which to operate. The report that follows represents a series of 50 patients with continued observation since the inception of the study in 1972, in which these principles were applied. All had been studied extensively and been declared totally disabled by independent opinions before being accepted for surgical treatment.

SURGICAL TECHNIQUE

The patient undergoing neural arch resection is premedicated routinely, according to the choice of the anesthesiologist. Endotracheal intubation is carried out with the administration of general anesthesia. An indwelling urinary catheter is inserted for fluid balance determinations during what may be a lengthy operative procedure. Intravascular lines are placed intravenously, intra-arterially, or both. The patient is positioned on bolsters on a surgical frame in the prone position, head slightly down, with care to leave the abdomen and chest free of ventral compression.

After surgical preparation and draping of the operative area, a midline lumbar incision is made and carried down through the superficial and deep fascia. The paraspinal musculature is reflected subperiosteally from the spinous processes, laminae, and facets, bilaterally. Hemostasis is achieved and neural arch resection is begun by removal of the spinous processes and laminae with rongeurs. The ligamentum flavum is removed and hemostasis of the epidural space is accomplished with cautery and cottonoid-Gelfoam* packing of the veins. For removal of the articulations, attention is directed to the side opposite the surgeon where the nerve root, foramen, and articular processes can best be identified. A flat probe is inserted into the foramen to assess the mobility of the nerve root and size of the foraminal canal. Sometimes this maneuver can be difficult when the edges of one or both processes are hypertrophied to approximate the floor of the canal or when lipping of the vertebral body has occurred with or without further encroachment by protrusion of the intervertebral disc. Removal of the medial edges of the facets will ease this maneuver. On occasion, this cannot be accomplished without undue risk to the nerve root so that resection of the inferior articular process may have to be carried out before the floor of the spinal canal can be visualized. When the nerve root and its axilla have been exposed, the floor is explored for extruded disc material which must then be removed. If the annulus has not been breached, no matter how much it may protrude, the disc is not violated and the bony dissection is carried forth.

Attention is now given to the intervertebral foramen and its overlying bony complex, consisting of the pars interarticularis, part of the pedicle, the inferior articular process, and superior articular process from the vertebral segment below. The soft tissue covering this complex is dissected free. The lateral edge is easily identified by meeting the dorsal lumbar artery, which may require bipolar coagulation for hemostasis. The medial edge of the pars and inferior articulation are rongeured away to the greatest extent possible using a flat-bottomed punch. The nerve root is under

direct vision ensuring its protection. When this maneuver has been carried as far laterally as space over the root will allow, the pars is rongeured directly using a Leksell rongeur from dorsal to ventral, carefully placing the opposing cups with their tips perpendicular to the floor. In this fashion, the pars can be thinned until it cracks, thereby avoiding instrumentation beneath it and the underlying entrapped root. Chisels are not used for this maneuver, thus lessening any risk of transmitted forces which may result in a traumatic neuritis or a contusion of the nerve root. With the pars broken, the capsule of the joint can be opened. The inferior articular process is lifted free and its base is removed to the pedicle. This exposes a length of the nerve root, usually including its ganglion, and it is now possible to follow its direction obliquely caudally and assess its relationship to the superior process extending upward from the spinal segment below. The superior aspect of the next lower root can be seen in proximity to the pedicle below entering the next lower foramen. To view this segment well may require removal of the medial edge of the superior articular process first, followed by the total removal of the process to the pedicle. Care must be exercised during the lateral dissection since the process here is in intimate relationship to the underlying obliquely placed nerve root which may be displaced posteriorly by a lateral protruding intervertebral disc. One-half of the neural arch resection has now been accomplished. The procedure is concluded by coagulation of the epidural veins and resection of fat, vascular pedicle, scar and, if the patient has had previous surgery, lysis of adhesions along the entire length of the nerve root until it turns ventrally to enter the retroperitoneal space. Should the nerve root not lie free and mobile in the spinal canal, as a consequence of a narrowly placed or thick pedicle, this structure is removed also. To complete the neural arch resection, the same technique is utilized on the contralateral side. To do

---

* Gelfoam, absorbable gelatin sponge, The Upjohn Co., Kalamazoo, MI.

so, the surgeon moves to the opposite side of the table, enhancing his visualization of the lateral aspects of the operative field.

When more than one level of resection is indicated, the same technique is accomplished at each additional segment. Final hemostasis is achieved with bipolar coagulation and Gelfoam. Inspection of the spinal canal is accomplished before closure to be certain the dural sac and all nerve roots are dissected free and lie clear of any bony encroachment. The appearance should be that of a "Christmas tree."

The area is covered with a layer of Gelfoam or fat as a deterrent to formation of postoperative adhesions. Copious irrigation is used and the incision is closed in layers using interrupted sutures. A drain may be utilized, according to surgical preference. No bony fusion is attempted. A firm dressing is applied across the lumbar area and out over the flanks. No supporting device is prescribed.

Postoperatively, the patient is left supine for 6 hours, then rotated side-back-side every 2 hours. Morphine is the preferred analgesic. Fluids and blood are replaced as indicated. The patient is mobilized the next day and re-enters a back rehabilitation program which was started preoperatively as conditioning for surgery.

PATIENT DATA

The 50 patients in this series ranged in age from the third to eighth decades of life; those in the fifth and sixth decades predominated. Women outnumbered men, 30 to 20, respectively.

Aside from low back pain, unilateral leg pain was present in the majority of the patients (30 of 50). Twelve patients had back and bilateral leg pain, five had leg pain alone, and three had back pain alone. This display of unilateral extension of pain, often localized to one defined root, could lead to the erroneous conclusion of single-level discogenic compression if history alone were the criterion.

The majority of patients had experienced pain for many years, 16 of the 50 for more than 10 years, one-half for more than 5 years. Only six patients complained of pain for less than 6 months. Long histories were the rule rather than the exception.

Of the 50 patients 14 had had no previous surgical treatment. The remaining 36 had undergone one or more surgical procedures.

As with pain, unilateral sensory or motor symptoms were present in the majority (28 of 50), once more erroneously suggesting single-level unilateral disease. It is of importance to note that 13 of the 50 patients had overt bladder symptoms, either retention or incomplete emptying. This is consistent with previously published data demonstrating neurogenic bladder dysfunction with compressive lesions of the lumbar spine.[11]

Bilateral sensory, motor, or reflex deficits were found in 27 of the 50 patients. The sharp reversal of laterality symptoms and signs is the key to the diagnosis of bony lesions of the lumbar spine. Not only were the findings bilateral, they were also multilevel. Twenty-one patients had unilateral deficits but they were often multisegmental. Only two patients had no detectable neurologic disturbance.

Mechanical signs such as the positive sciatic stretch signs or evoked extension of radicular pain on back range of motion were found less frequently. Of the 50 patients, 27 had no positive findings, none were bilaterally positive, and 14 were unilaterally significant. Again, the hallmarks of single root compression were not prominent, suggestive of other pathology.

DIAGNOSTIC TESTS

Among those patients who underwent electromyography, 17 of 24 patients with positive studies had bilateral or multilevel abnormalities. Only seven patients had unilateral, single-level changes. This was an important adjunct to the neurologic examination in the effort to detect any evidence of multiple root disturbance.

Standard lumbosacral radiographs were found to be strongly positive when reviewed discriminately for those changes seen with lumbar stenosis (Table 6.1). Of the 50 patients, 16 had diagnoses on plain films of frank stenosis. Facet hypertrophy was the most common abnormality. There were 15 patients with spondylolisthesis, eight of whom had the degenerative form. Congenital anomalies, other than olisthesis, were found in 11 patients. Multiple-level disease was again prominent in 33 of the 50 patients.

Computerized axial tomography was carried out in 47 of the 50 patients (Table 6.2). All but two had demonstrable disease. Stenosis was confirmed in 29 patients, with facet hypertrophy providing the major deformities. Fusion ingrowth was seen in four instances. Arch asymmetry was found with or without accompanying facetal hypertrophy. Again, multiple levels of involvement were demonstrated in 27 of the 47 patients.

Myelography disclosed stenosis in 28 of 44 patients in whom studies were done (Table 6.3). Despite the history of previous surgery, multiple in more than one-half of

Table 6.1. Standard lumbosacral radiographs

Stenosis	16
Facet hypertrophy	32
Spondylolisthesis, degenerative	8
Spondylolisthesis, congenital	7
Transitional vertebra	5
Arch anomaly	6
Compression fracture	1
Normal	2
Missing	2
Multiple levels	33

Table 6.2. Computerized axial tomography

Facet hypertrophy	33
Stenosis	29
Fusion ingrowth	4
Arch assymetry	5
Normal	2
Not done	3
Multiple levels	27

Table 6.3. Pantopaque myelography

Stenosis	28
Lateral defect	3
Posterior defect	16
Hour glass deformity	8
Ventral defect	9
Narrow dural sac	2
Epidural scar	5
Arachnoiditis	1
Meningocele, diverticulum	3
Normal	1
Not done	6
Multiple levels	21

36 patients, significant epidural scarring or arachnoiditis was thought to be present in only six patients. Therefore, the description of this entity, so often seen in operative notes of "failed back surgery," is not the issue; bony encroachment is. Once more, multiple-level disease was common.

RESULTS

The 50 patients in this series underwent 110 neural arch resections. Only 10 patients had single arch removals; 23 were double, 15 triple, one four- and one five-level. The outcome was classified into five functional groups. Group I comprises patients free from pain who have returned to full activity, including work. Patients in Group II are at full activity with some pain but no medication. Patients in Group III are moderately restricted, perform acts of daily living, but may take non-narcotic analgesics. Those in Group IV are severely restricted, may require narcotics, and have a sedentary existence. Group V patients remain totally disabled. Better results were achieved in those patients who had multilevel surgery, again suggesting the principle that all diseased segments must be corrected if return of function without pain is to be attained. One-half of this group who were totally disabled preoperatively have regained a normal to nearly normal existence and have maintained this state during the follow-up period, ranging up to 7 years. There were 19 compensation cases among those groups. The results in the compensation cases cannot be distinguished from the noncompensation cases suggesting that it is the manner of treatment, not the corporate structure or socioeconomic aspect of the case, which is important to outcome.

COMPLICATIONS

The most troublesome complication for this group of 110 patients who underwent neural arch resections was infection: two were superficial and four were deep, presumably because of the large dead space left in the wound allowing serum collection and ease of contamination. All were controlled without untoward consequences. Three patients required prolonged continuous or intermittent catheterization programs, however, it must be noted that each had a neurogenic bladder preoperatively. One patient had hepatitis, one had a pulmonary embolism, and one had paresis, but all recovered. Olisthesis did occur in one patient, but subluxation was secondary to another traumatic event. The immediate resulting symptoms were managed conservatively and stabilization was not considered to be an issue. Fusion was not performed, symptoms remitted, and no further slip occurred. Finally, there were no deaths in this series.

DISCUSSION

This chapter is not intended to describe a single operative procedure to answer all surgical questions concerning lumbar spinal spondylosis or stenosis. Rather, it describes an adapted technique born of years of frustration and limited success in a difficult field. The evaluation of the surgical technique was made possible by the development of axial radiology, and definitive precise viewing of the spinal column which demonstrates the clear-cut role of bony encroachment as a source of lumbar disability. As a consequence, there is a growing realization that the herniated intervertebral disc is not the sole offending pathologic factor.

Further, the indiscriminate removal of disc material, which is capable of providing only a limited restoration of intraspinal reserve, is to be decried. Enlargement of the canal, particularly where it is required laterally beneath the articular processes, is an absolute necessity. This is an anatomic domain which heretofore has not been delineated well by clinical examination, diagnostic adjuncts, or direct observation in the operating theater. Moreover, central laminectomy will not correct lateral stenosis, a disease of the lateral articular processes.

Neural arch resection involves two principles of application. Bony encroachments of stenotic degree must be removed in their entirety at the level of involvement. Each diseased level, however many there may be, must be treated concurrently. Thus, one or all lumbar segments may require resection and a simple laminectomy will not suffice. Whether or not neural arch resection produces mechanical instability remains a question not yet fully answered. After 7 years of application, instability secondary to this procedure does not appear to be an issue. The one case of nonprogressive olisthesis in this series conforms with the published incidence of 2% of conventional, less radical surgery.[12] Therefore, spinal fusion has not been carried out since instability or progression of the uncommon olisthesis has yet to be demonstrated.[13]

Patients become candidates for neural arch resection when all modalities of conservative management have failed to provide lasting benefit. If previous disc surgery has been unsuccessful, undetected bony encroachment has been the usual cause. Therefore, neural arch resection should have been the primary procedure when stenosis or its elements can be demonstrated objectively. Special mention of pseudo-spondylolisthesis, also called degenerative or acquired spondylolisthesis, should be made. Its recognition is important since relief of pain is rarely achieved without surgery. This is in contradistinction to congenital spondylolisthesis which will respond to nonsurgical methods in many instances.

Results of neural arch resection indicate a full return of function to one-half of its recipients who, in this series, were totally disabled before surgery. Another one-fourth regained capacity to perform acts of daily living, although some pain persisted. The remaining one-fourth continue disabled, however, it is hoped that they will still improve. The last statement is predicated on the observation that neural arch resection results seem to improve with time, especially if the patient maintains the postoperative rehabilitation conditioning program to which they agree as a condition for entering this treatment mode. These results are equal in compensation and noncompensation cases.

Despite the extent of the surgical procedure, complications are few. Infection has been the most prevalent although less so in the more recent cases. Postoperative spondylolisthesis or instability has not been a problem, as indicated previously.

SUMMARY

A series of 50 patients with lumbar spondylosis or stenosis who have undergone the procedure of neural arch resection has been presented. The patients were predominantly in the fifth and sixth decades of life. Females outnumbered males three to two. Long histories and previous surgical treatment were characteristic with unilateral symptoms predominating. However, physical examination demonstrated the reverse, i.e., bilateral signs and multisegmental disease. Lumbosacral radiographs suggested a stenotic condition and myelography was corroborative. The definitive test was computed axial tomography. Neural arch resection removes, bilaterally, the spinous processes, laminae, articular processes, and the pedicles if the latter are hypertrophied or narrowly placed. Resection must be accomplished at all levels of disease for optimal results. Fusion has not been required.

One-half of a group of 50 totally disabled patients have returned to full function and comfort, one-fourth to performing acts of daily living with some pain, and one-fourth remaining disabled. Complications include six infections and one case of postoperative spondylolisthesis.

Neural arch resection is a procedure for the management of lumbar spondylosis or stenosis and its elemental categories. The results indicate at least a 50% expectation of return to function in comfort provided that the principles of surgery as to extent and removal of disease at all levels are followed and that the patients participate in a back rehabilitation and conditioning program.

References

1. Kirkaldy-Willis, W. H., McIvor, G. W. D.: Spinal stenosis. *Clin. Orthopaed.* 115:2, 1976.
2. LaRocca, H., McNab, I.: The laminectomy membrane. *J. Bone Joint Surg.* 56B:545, 1974.
3. Weinstein, P. R., Ehni, G., Wilson, C. B.: *Lumbar Spondylosis.* Chicago, IL, Year Book Medical Publishers, Inc., 1977.
4. Gargano, F. P., Jacobson, R. E., Rosomoff, H. L.: Transverse axial radiology of the spine. *Neuroradiology* 6:254, 1974.
5. Jacobson, R. E., Gargano, R. P., Rosomoff, H. L.: Transverse axial tomography of the spine. Part 1. Axial anatomy of the normal lumbar spine. *J. Neurosurg.* 42:406, 1975.
6. Jacobson, R. E., Gargano, F. P., Rosomoff, H. L.: Transverse axial tomography of the spine. Part 2. The stenotic spinal canal. *J. Neurosurg.* 42:412, 1975.
7. Post, M. J. D., Gargano, F. P., Vining, D. Q., Rosomoff, H. L.: A comparison of radiographic methods of diagnosing constructive lesions of the spinal canal. Toshiba unit vs CT scanner. *J. Neurosurg.* 48:360, 1978.
8. Rosomoff, H. L., Post, J. D., Quencer, R. M.: Axial radiology of the lumbar spine. *Clin. Neurosurg.* 25:251, 1978.
9. Gill, G. G., Manning, J. G., White, H. L.: Surgical treatment of spondylolisthesis without spine fusion. *J. Bone Joint Surg.* 37A:493, 1955.
10. Rosomoff, H. L.: Bony encroachment of the lumbar spine. A cause of low back surgery failure. *J. Fla. Med. Assoc.* 63:884, 1976.
11. Rosomoff, H. L., Johnston, J. D. H., Gallo, A. E., Ludmer, M., Givens, F. T., Carney, F. T., Keuhn, C. A.: Cystometry as an adjunct in the evaluation of lumbar disc syndromes. *J. Neurosurg.* 33:67, 1970.
12. Hanraets, O.: *The Degenerative Back and its Differential Diagnosis.* New York, NY, Elsevier Publishing Co., 1959.
13. White, A. H., Wiltse, L. L.: *Post-operative Spondylolisthesis in Lumbar Spondylosis.* Chicago, IL, Year Book Medical Publishers, Inc., 1977, p. 184.

7

Posterior Lumbar Interbody Fusion

The concept of intervertebral (intercorporeal) fusion in the cervical area has gained wide acceptance in recent years. In 1945, Cloward[1] devised "The treatment of ruptured lumbar disc by intervertebral fusion—report of 100 cases" and first reported at the Harvey Cushing Society meeting at Hot Springs, Virginia, in November 1947. His description of the technique of posterior lumbar interbody fusion predated by 12 years his more popular cervical anterior fusion. With the exception of Cloward's own publications,[2, 3] there has been astonishingly little enthusiasm for posterior lumbar interbody fusion.

The practice of posterior lumbar interbody fusion is more popular outside the United States. Crock[4] of Australia indicates that the ideal operation for isolated lumbar disc resorption (localized spondylosis) is the posterior lumbar interbody fusion. LeVay[5] of England reports that the posterior lumbar interbody fusion is favored by neurosurgeons there. Junghanns and Schmorl[6] of Germany are advocates of Cloward's concept of the posterior lumbar interbody fusion. Junghanns believes that the unstable lumbar segments should not only be fused, but should also effect an operative unfolding (*distraction*) of the disc space. "In the lumbar spine this only could be achieved posteriorly by removing disc tissue, eliminating the cartilaginous plate, unfolding (*distraction*) of the disc space, and positioning of the osseous packs," Junghanns concluded. (Italics are the author's). Wiltberger,[7, 8] is also in favor of posterior lumbar interbody fusion. He modifies the technique by insertion of dowel grafts instead of peg grafts. Wiltberger inserts the dowel grafts through the facet without prior dissection or isolation of the nerve root.

In discussing posterior lumbar interbody fusion, there are two principles that should be brought into focus:

The first is the concept that the lumbar intervertebral disc is a part of the motion segment (Fig. 7.1). Junghanns and Schmorl[6] were the first to describe it as only part of the motor segment or perhaps better translated as motion segment (*bewegungssegment*). The motion segment also consists of intervertebral disc, intervertebral foramen, facet, interlaminal space, ligamentum flavum, spinous processes, and adjoining ligaments. Junghanns' concept is that with a change in the disc space, there is also an associated change in all of the motion segments. When a lumbar disc is degenerative or if the disc is removed surgically, the intervertebral disc space will settle and the narrowing is followed with sequential changes in the motion segment as a whole (Fig. 7.2). There would be, in addition to disc herniation, posterior spur formation of the vertebral body, facet overriding, spur formation of the facet, or internal invagination of ligamentum flavum. In various combinations, the result is neural compression at various sections of the spinal segment. Spinal stenosis, both of the intervertebral foramen and the spinal canal, often follows simple discectomy with subsequent disc space settling after surgery.

The next principle is tropism, defined as a nonmotile organismatic response elicited by an external stimulus. It is also described as the turning or movement of protoplasm

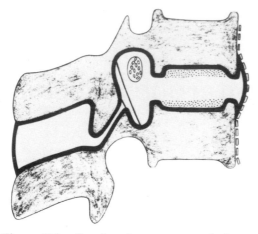

Figure 7.1. Junghann's concept of *bewegungssegment* "motor segment" or "motion segment" with disc and facet working as a single motion unit. Note the ligamentum flavum covering the anterior portion of the facet.

Tropism, of course, can be seen in computed tomographic (CT) scans (Fig. 7.5). However, in the absence of this method,

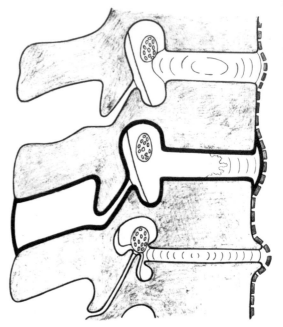

Figure 7.2. Sequential changes expected in a motor segment when the disc material is extruded or removed surgically. Laterally ligamentum flavum lies anterior to the facet and is generally not radiologically identifiable.

or organized matter. This description, as applied to the facet or apophyseal joint, indicates inversion or hypertrophy of the facet joint. This change is due to excessive or abnormal external stimulation which is related to motion or static stress of the facet from an abnormal motion segment. Hypertrophic arthrosis of the facet or inversion of the facet joint is, therefore, the result of abnormal external or static stress on the facet, related to motion (Fig. 7.3).

Tropism is the primary cause of lateral spinal stenosis. Lateral spinal stenosis at one level would compress two pairs of intervertebral nerves (Fig. 7.4).

(1) *Narrow lateral spinal recess* results in subarticular entrapment of the nerve root, leaving the intervertebral foramen at the next inferior level.

(2) *Foraminal stenosis* is the result of settling of the disc space, spur formation, and overriding of the facets. The result is impingement of the nerve root against the pedicle at the same level. If surgery is designed to remove the effects of the tropism of the facet joint, total arrest of the motion by fusion is a prerequisite to prevent recurrent trophic changes of the facet.

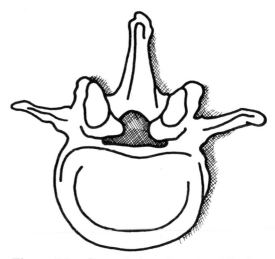

Figure 7.3. Coronal view of tropism: The hypertrophic arthrosis and tropism of the posterior joints are mainly responsible for a localized spinal stenosis.

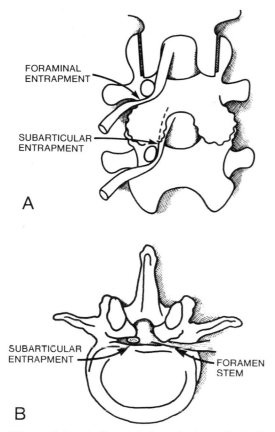

FORAMINAL
ENTRAPMENT

SUBARTICULAR
ENTRAPMENT

A

SUBARTICULAR
ENTRAPMENT

FORAMEN
STEM

B

Figure 7.4. A. Coronal view of a lateral spinal stenosis showing hypertrophy and tropism of the facet producing: (a) subarticular compression of the nerve leaving the level below and (b) foraminal compression of the nerve leaving at the same level. B. Anteroposterior (AP) view of a lateral spinal stenosis at one level showing compression of two pairs of intervertebral nerves. Foraminal compression of the nerve leaving the same level above the disc space and subarticular entrapment of the nerve leaving the foramen below.

the diagnosis can still be confirmed by recognition of a facet cleft on true lateral view (Fig. 7.6) and a long lateral defect on myelogram (Fig. 7.7). Having made a decision that fusion may be desirable, the following advantages of posterior lumbar interbody fusion (PLIF) should be considered.

(1) PLIF reconstitutes the normal anatomic relationship between the motion segment and the neural structures. The narrow disc space and the motion segment are restored to normal anatomic alignment.

(2) Successful PLIF would arrest further degenerative process of the fused motion segment. However, because of an increased range of motion of the adjoining vertebral disc spaces, their degenerative processes could be enhanced by PLIF.

(3) Total discectomy needed for PLIF would prevent recurrent lumbar disc herniation at that level.

(4) PLIF would prevent painful nerve irritation from postoperative perineural adhesions. Lack of motion after a successful PLIF would prevent mechanical pulling of the nerve root by the surrounding scar tissue.

(5) Wide laminotomy in PLIF relieves all neural compression, especially in cases of lateral spinal stenosis.

(6) PLIF restores a constant relationship between all the components of a motion segment. It also prevents tropism of the facet.

INDICATIONS FOR PLIF

Keim[9] has listed ten indications for lumbar spine fusion, with which we concur. These are:

(1) unstable joint complex associated with a long history of low back pain;

(2) spondylolisthesis with or without spondylolysis;

(3) congenital anomaly, transitional transverse process, or spondylolysis without spondylolisthesis;

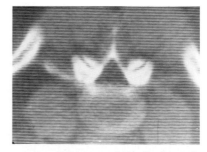

Figure 7.5. CT scan of L5-S1 lateral spinal stenosis showing giant bulbous hypertrophy of the facet eliminating the lateral recesses.

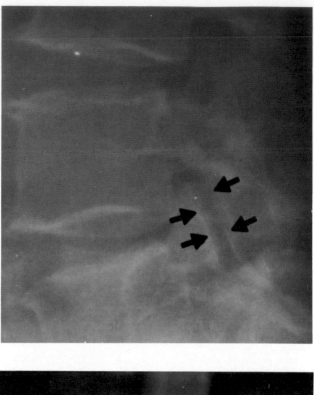

Figure 7.6. Lateral radiogram showing a clear-cut facet joint indicating that the joint is coronal in orientation—tropism.

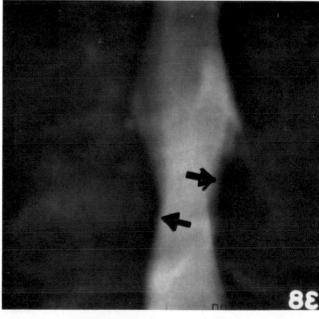

Figure 7.7. AP myelogram of the lumbar spine. Long lateral defects are due to dorsal and lateral compression of the whole length of the coronal oriented facet joint.

(4) localized lateral spinal stenosis or degenerative spondylosis at one level;

(5) facet resection from previous surgery;

(6) heavy labor or sports activity associated with simple disc herniation with or without degenerative change;

(7) bilateral disc herniation or massive midline herniation;

CLOWARD'S PLIF

PROBLEMS	SOLUTIONS
1. Visibility	1. Fiberoptic lighting
2. Hemostasis	2. a. Position of patient b. Surgicel tamponade c. Bipolar coagulation
3. Instability—facet resection	3. Mesial facectomy
4. Settlement and angulation— removal of cortical plates	4. Robinson's principle Preservation of cortical plate
5. Failure of osteosynthesis	5. a. Autogenous grafts b. Generous cancellous bone grafts mixed with cortical peg grafts c. Compression—Unipour concept d. Knight's lumbar brace—four months

Figure 7.8. Problems and solutions of Cloward's original posterior lumbar interbody fusion technique.

(8) previous disc surgery at that level;

(9) reconstruction for failed back surgery syndrome (FBSS), including pseudoarthrodesis from lateral fusion;

(10) obese patients with laterally extruded discs—prevention of rapid postoperative settling of the disc space.

TECHNIQUE

Potential problems of Cloward's original PLIF were studied and solutions formulated (Fig. 7.8). A modification[10] of Cloward's posterior lumbar interbody fusion is introduced with the following characteristics:

(1) A better technique of controlling epidural hemorrhage was developed by emphasizing the lessening of the epidural venous pressure through proper positioning of the patient.

(2) Surgicel* was used in the form of tampons to control epidural bleeding, thus avoiding the excessive use of electric coagulation of the epidural venous plexus.

_____

* Surgicel. Oxidised cellulose, Johnson & Johnson, New Brunswick, New Jersey.

(3) The integrity of the facet was preserved through a more limited interlaminal approach.

(4) The cortical plate was preserved and osteosynthesis of the graft assured by multiple perforations of the cortical plate in accordance with Robinson's[11, 12] principle as applied to anterior cervical interbody fusion.

Illumination

Excellent illumination is critical to the success of this procedure. We routinely use a fiber optic headlight.

Position

The position of the patient is prone (Fig. 7.9). The rolls used to support the patient must be firm and customized to fit the patient's height and weight. They must be placed laterally so that the inferior vena cava and the femoral veins are not compressed. The pressure points should be at the clavicle, ribs, and anterior iliac crest. The surgeon must place his hands between the rolls after the patient is placed on the table to be sure that the anterior abdominal

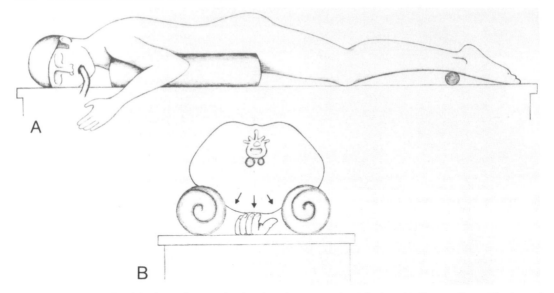

Figure 7.9. A. Positioning of posterior lumbar intervertebral fusion. Rolls are firm. Flexion of table not needed. B. Testing the tension of anterior abdominal wall.

wall is suspended freely. There must be no undue pressure on the inferior vena cava. Many commercially available rolls have a slanting surface which will compress the inferior vena cava through the lateral compression on the abdominal wall. The table is not flexed; flexing the table increases the intra-abdominal venous pressure, thus increasing epidural hemorrhage. It also could increase the incidence of thrombophlebitis from venous stagnation in the lower extremities.

Incision

The incision is horizontal (Fig. 7.10). Grafts can be removed from the posterior iliac crest through the same incision. Three disc levels can be explored through this horizontal approach.

Exposure

The usual bilateral laminotomy exposure is used (Fig. 7.11). The amount of bone removed is no more than for an ordinary decompressive laminotomy done for cauda equina compression. The medial half of the facet is chiseled away by a sharp osteotome to gain exposure just lateral to the nerve

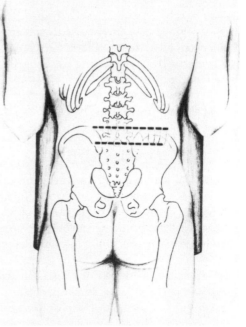

Figure 7.10. Incision for posterior lumbar intervertebral fusion. *Upper dotted line* is for L4–5 disc and *lower dotted line* is for L5-S1 disc.

root. Total removal of the facet could produce postoperative instability resulting in spondylolisthesis.

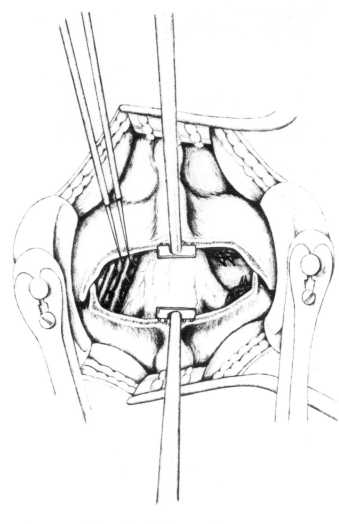

Figure 7.11. Bilateral laminotomy with preservation of the facets. Control of epidural hemorrhage. Bipolar or insulted coagulation forceps are used on the *left side*. On the *right side*, epidural hemorrhage is controlled by impacted Surgicel tampons. Impacted Surgicel tampons also push the nerve root medially and expose the disc space without the need of nerve root retractor.

In cases of lateral spinal stenosis, a medial facetectomy would relieve the nerve impinged by subarticular entrapment (Fig. 7.12). The true foraminotomy for foraminal stenosis would require the amputation of the upper portion of the superior facet, and this can be accomplished by angular punch, angular curette, small osteotome, or Sonic curette (25000 c.p.s.).† (Fig. 7.13). This is in distinct contrast to the conventional foraminotomy where the superior laminae are unroofed over the nerve leaving the foramen of the space below (Figs. 7.4, 7.13, and 7.14).

---

† Manufactured by Quintron, Inc., P.O. Box 562, Worthington, Ohio 43085.

A strong functioning posterior supraspinous ligament must be preserved. This would add to the stability of the graft (Fig. 7.15).

Epidural Hemostasis

The success of this operation depends on mastering the technique of controlling epidural hemorrhage. A prerequisite is the proper positioning of the patient so that the venous pressure within the epidural space is reduced to a minimum. Surgicel is used as a tampon to control epidural bleeding (Fig. 7.11). The epidural veins can be cut with scissors and then pushed out of the way with a ball or tampon of Surgicel above

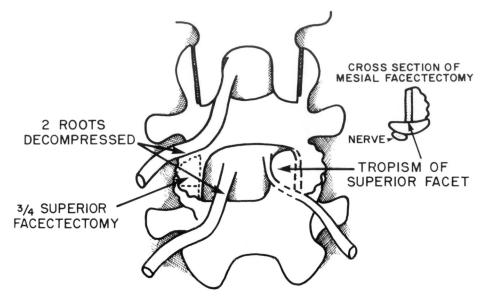

Figure 7.12. AP view showing that in PLIF the mesial facectectomy does relieve subarticular nerve compression.

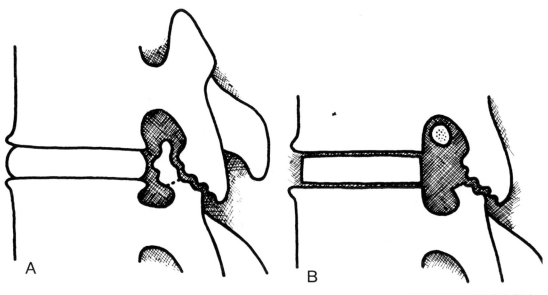

FORAMINAL STENOSIS PLIF FORAMINOTOMY

Figure 7.13. Lateral view of an encroached intervertebral foramen (A). "True" foraminotomy is accomplished by partial facectectomy, especially the superior facet (B).

and below the disc space. The bleeding, of course, could be controlled by coagulation (Fig. 7.11), preferably bipolar. Generally, the veins are longitudinal. Sectioning of one or two longitudinal veins after coagulation

and then pushing the remaining veins out of the field with the Surgicel tampon makes the control of epidural bleeding a reasonably simple procedure. If the venous pressure within the epidural space is minimal,

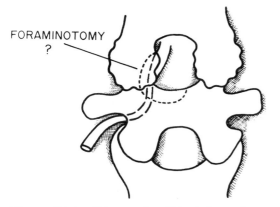

FORAMINOTOMY
?

Figure 7.14. "Conventional" technique of unroofing upper laminae is NOT a foraminotomy.

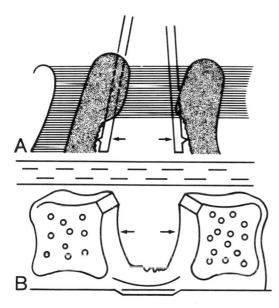

PRESERVATION OF THE POSTERIOR INTERSPINOUS LIGAMENTS

Figure 7.15. Preservation of posterior portion of the supraspinous ligament would enhance: (A) avoidance of postoperative flexion injury which may dislodge the grafts; (B) locking mechanism during laminal distraction procedure and a more even distraction of the emptied disc space.

the bleeding can be controlled without using coagulation. Bleeding from the lateral gutter can also be controlled by impacting a smaller piece of Surgicel into this area.

On very rare occasions, there is a small amount of arterial bleeding which does require careful bipolar coagulation and, if necessary, the help of a magnification device. The Surgicel tampon would also retract the dura and the nerve root medially. With the use of such tampons, the prolonged use of metallic nerve root retractors can be avoided. This is a definite advantage in minimizing nerve root injury. The laminal retractor is used to distract the disc space for better exposure and, when it is removed after the grafts have been inserted, compression of the grafts is enhanced. The laminal retractor should be used just before insertion of the graft. For reasons not totally apparent, we found that when the laminal retractor is applied and the laminae are distracted forcibly, there may be an increase in epidural bleeding. We, therefore, use the laminal retractor at the completion of the total discectomy just before insertion of the grafts.

Discectomy

The adjoining intervertebral rims are first chiseled away (Fig. 7.16). This accomplishes three objectives: it enlarges the en-

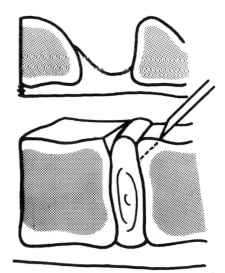

Figure 7.16. Before attempts are made to radically remove the disc material, the intervertebral rims are first chiseled away.

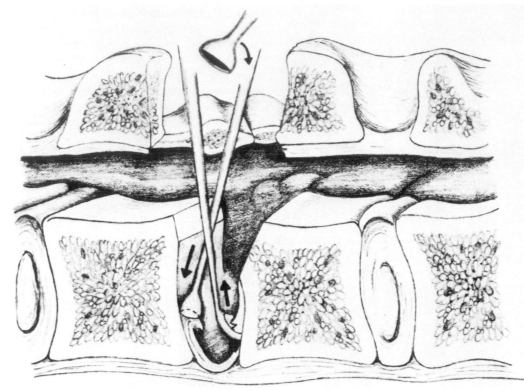

Figure 7.17. After the intervertebral rims are removed, identify the cleavage of disc attachment to cortical plate and use downbite or upbite currette energetically to detach the disc materials from the cortical plate. Curved upbite currette is used to remove the concaved centrum of the lower cartilaginous plate. Then remove the detached large chunks of disc material with a ronguer.

trance to the disc space, it exposes the cancellous bone posteriorly, and it exposes a cleavage between the cartilaginous plate and the cortical bone.

After the cortical plate is exposed, all disc material and the cartilaginous plate are removed energetically by sharp curetting and rongeuring with either upbite or downbite instrumentation. The centrum of the lower cortical plate often is slightly concave so that the cartilaginous material can be removed only by a curved upbite curette (Fig. 7.17). Total discectomy is needed before the disc space is ready to receive the grafts.

Next, any midline bar must be removed (Fig. 7.18). This could be difficult. The annulus should be separated from the posterior longitudinal ligament with Cloward's cervical periosteal elevator and then pushed downward with a right angle down-

bite curette. Often, the midline bar only can be removed after it has been pushed by a medially advanced graft.

Graft Site Preparation

The cortical plate then is penetrated at many points. The use of chisel alone is not effective. To make larger and deeper penetrations into the cancellous bone, Cloward's cervical periosteal elevator can be modified to use as a perforator (Fig. 7.19). This instrument is sharp pointed and has a 45° angulation. Downward tapping of this instrument should result in horizontal entrance into the cancellous bone. Radical perforation of the cortical plate would facilitate revascularization of the grafts. In effect, we are utilizing Robinson's cervical interbody principle in Cloward's posterior lumbar interbody fusion. The preservation

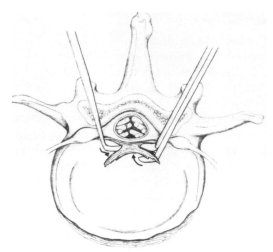

Figure 7.18. Removal of midline bar of annulus fibrosus. Sharp-pointed osteophyte periosteal elevator is used to separate the disc material from posterior limiting membrane and then removed by either a sharp angled upbite disc ronguer or "peapod" pituitary ronguer.

of the cortical plate is important to avoid settling. If the cortical plate is thick and sclerotic, it is advisable to remove part of the cortical plate by a rotation action of a large and sharp curette (1–2 mm. larger than the disc space) or a sonic curette.

Graft Removal

A split-thickness graft is then removed from the iliac bone posteriorly. The graft removed is about 8 mm thick, 3–5 cm wide, and 6–8 cm long (Fig. 7.20). The graft is then removed en bloc by using an osteotome. Six to eight generous strips of cancellous bone are removed to fit the available space distally and laterally in the prepared bed after total discectomy. The en bloc graft then is cut into widths depending on the height of the disc space after it is totally distracted. A power saw is used for the preparation of the grafts. Each graft is gen-

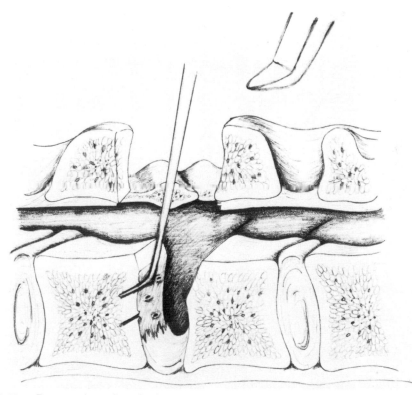

Figure 7.19. Preparation of graft site—osteotomy of the epiphyseal ring, preservation of the cortical plate, and penetration of cortical plate to enhance revascularization of grafts from the cancellous bone.

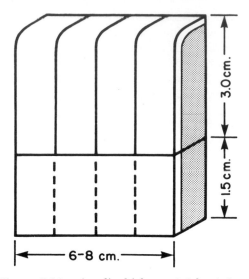

Figure 7.20. A split thickness 6–8 by 4–5 cm en bloc graft is removed from the posterior iliac crest. The graft is long enough to have four extra half-length peg grafts.

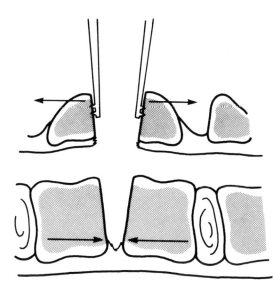

Figure 7.21. Laminal retractor would distract the laminae but the leverage action of the motion segment actually may narrow the disc space distally, making it difficult to receive a rectangular peg graft.

erally about 10 mm in width and about 30 mm in length. If only four grafts can be obtained, four extra half-grafts can be procured by making the grafts deeper or wider.

Graft Insertion

The laminal retractor may not be effective in distracting the distal disc space (Fig. 7.21). Insertion of Cloward's impactor deep into the disc space, with leverage action, may give a larger disc space entrance to the initial central graft. The prying distraction can be repeated on the other side to facilitate the insertion of the several central grafts (Fig. 7.22). If the disc space is not large enough to admit a vertebral body retractor, this may be preferable to the lamina retractor. The vertebral body retractor only can be used on one side; a lamina retractor may or may not be needed for graft insertion of the opposite disc space.

Before the peg grafts are inserted, the depth of the disc space is filled with one to two strips of cancellous bone. The peg grafts are then inserted with the cortical bone of the graft along the longitudinal axis of the body. With the disc space fully distracted by the laminal retractor (vertebral body retractor) or by deeply inserting Cloward's Puka impactor, the grafts can be pushed into the disc space with only a slight tapping. A slight swiveling movement of the blunt end of the chisel (Puka impactor)

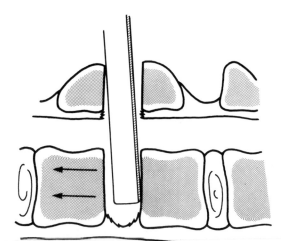

Figure 7.22. Insert the Cloward impactor to the depth of the disc space and pry forcibly. This would distract the disc space evenly. A large medial graft can be inserted into the opposite side and then reverse the process.

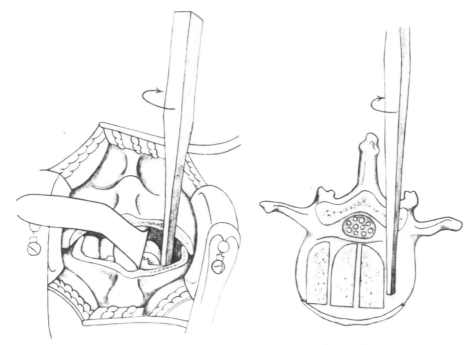

Figure 7.23. Medial graft advancement with single chisel.

will move the graft to the center so that a second graft can be placed laterally on the same side (Fig. 7.23).

If the graft is firmly impacted into the disc space, Cloward's Puka maneuver (medial displacement) may be needed to propel the first graft to the center. This technique entails using two blunt-end chisels and swiveling one against the other. At least four grafts are used, but six grafts are preferred. We fully agree with Cloward's teaching to "pack them tight" (Fig. 7.24). At least 50% of the disc space should be filled with grafts in order to avoid failure of osteosynthesis (Fig. 7.25). Also, we have been placing cancellous bone strips in the lateral aspect of the disc space. All crevices between the peg grafts should be filled with cancellous bone (Fig. 7.26). We firmly believe that a tightly impacted disc space with many cancellous and peg grafts is essential to the success of the fusion. The normal weight bearing of the adjoining vertebral bodies results in a natural locking mechanism for the grafts.

When the intervertebral foramen is well decompressed through the medial facetectomy of the superior facet, the nerve root that leaves the foramen of the same level is very close to the lateral margin of the disc space. This nerve root often can be seen after the decompression. When the lateralmost graft is impacted, the graft may split, displace laterally, and impinge on this nerve root (Fig. 7.27). After all grafts are inserted, care must be taken that no undue pressure from the grafts is exerted on the nerve root that is in front and easily visible. Also, a search should be conducted for any possible bony impingement of the lateral nerve root which is behind and often partially hidden.

Closure

The Surgicel is removed at the end of the procedure and epidural bleeding is controlled with Gelfoam.‡ The donor site bleeding can be easily controlled with Gel-

---

‡ Gelfoam. Absorbable gelatine sponge, The Upjohn Co., Kalamazoo, Michigan.

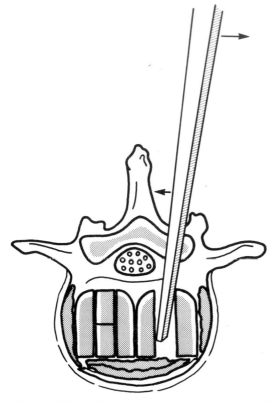

Figure 7.24. Six peg grafts. Two are one-half length peg grafts. The disc space is very tightly packed. Cancellous bone grafts are used to fill the spaces in depth and lateral recesses of the disc space.

foam soaked with Thrombin.§ There is no need to use a drain. Intraoperative Keflin‖ can be given 2 gm intravenously and continued at 2 gm every 6 hours for four doses. The average blood loss is between 200 and 400 cc, therefore transfusions rarely are necessary.

Postoperative Care

Patients should be out of bed in 2 or 3 days with a Knight's lumbar spinal brace. The timing of the ambulation can be judged by the ease with which the patients can

§ Thrombin. Topical (bovine origin), Parke-Davis, Division of Warner-Lambert Co., Morris Plains, New Jersey.

‖ Keflin. Cephalothin sodium. Eli Lilly & Co., Indianapolis, Indiana.

move themselves in bed. Many patients who previously have had simple discectomies claim that the pain from the posterior lumbar interbody fusion is less than that from simple discectomy. Generally, a solid fusion should occur within 4 months after surgery (Figs. 7.28–7.30). Depending on the result of tomograms done 4 months postoperatively, a decision can be made as to when the brace should be removed. Patients are encouraged to engage in any physical exercise within the confines of the Knight's lumbar spinal brace during the recuperative period.

Complications

The first 300 cases done by the author have shown no postoperative wound infection. There were six cases of postoperative thrombophlebitis, four occurred during the hospital stay with two occurring after discharge. There were six cases of increased neurologic deficit, manifested in a foot drop, which recovered between 6 weeks and 6 months after surgery. If, during surgery, a

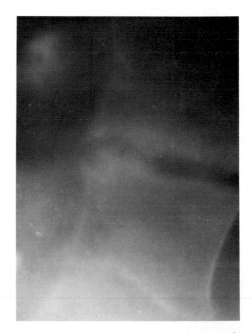

Figure 7.25. Pseudoarthrodesis occurs when the graft occupies less than the posterior 50% of the disc space.

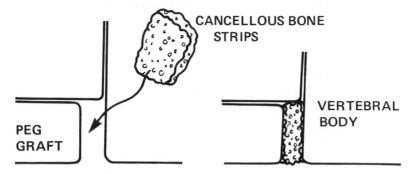

**FILL ALL CREVICES WITH CANCELLOUS BONE STRIPS
LIKE DENTAL FILLING OF CAVITIES**

Figure 7.26. Filling crevices between the peg grafts and vertebral body with cancellous bone grafts.

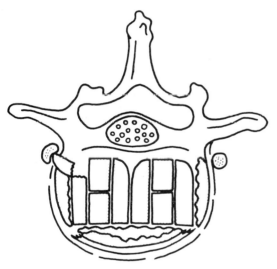

Figure 7.27. Schematic drawing showing the danger of the lateralmost graft broken, displaced, and impinging on the nerve behind the facet at the same level.

spinal fluid leakage is encountered, the leakage should be closed with suturing. If a water-tight closure is not possible, then the leakage should be controlled by Gelfoam or a muscle graft and the patient should be put on complete bed rest for 14 days before ambulation. In our series, we have not encountered any difficulty with cerebrospinal fluid leakage.

Most patients had mild discomfort at the donor site. About 7% had transient numbness over the anterior thigh in the distri-bution of the lateral femoral cutaneous nerve, secondary to compression of the nerve by the firm rolls used to support the body.

Results

Of a total series of 300 cases, 50 consecutive patients who were operated on, with at least a 24-month follow-up, were studied by two Board certified orthopaedic surgeons as to the success of the fusion and clinical improvement. Letters were sent out to all 50 patients inviting them to return for examination by the follow-up orthopaedic surgeons. Forty-five patients returned for examination. Of the patients examined, 31 were male, 14 were female. The male ages varied from 20–60 with an average of 42.1 years. The female ages varied from 20–60 with an average of 42.8 (Fig. 7.31A and B).

Of the 45 patients examined, 30 patients had surgery performed in L4–5 level, 14 had surgery in L5-S1 level, and one patient had surgery at both L3–4 and L4–5 levels (Fig. 7.32).

The clinical results are rated as:

(1) excellent—complete recovery, resuming normal activity, not on medication.

(2) good—returned to work, occasional mild analgesic, enjoying work and recreation.

(3) fair—works under duress, takes oc-

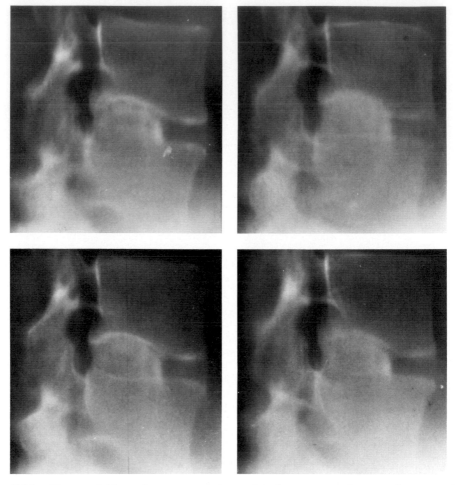

Figure 7.28. Four serial lateral tomograms, 4 months after surgery, show good osteosynthesis in all cuts.

casional medication, better than before surgery.

(4) poor—needs medication in a dependent fashion, unable to return to work, denied any improvement.

In this series, none claimed they were worse than before the surgery.

Thirty-seven of the patients or 82% had radiologic fusion. This was demonstrated either by tomogram or flexion extension lateral film or both. Two had questionable fusion. Pseudoarthrodesis occurred in six patients or 13.3% (Fig. 7.33).

The clinical result was rated as excellent in 25 patients (55.5%) and good result was obtained in 6 patients (13.3%) giving a total

satisfactory group, comprised of patients reporting excellent and good results, of 68.8% (Fig. 7.34A). Fair result occurred in 7 patients (15.5%) and poor result also occurred in 7 patients (15.5%). Fourteen patients (31.2%) had less than satisfactory result. In this group, there were 11 documented problem patients with secondary gain (compensation or litigation). Only one had excellent result, four had fair result, and six had poor result.

If one is to eliminate the patients who had secondary gain, then excellent to good result would be elevated to 88.2% in contrast to 68.8% (Fig. 7.34B).

In the excellent group, only one had a

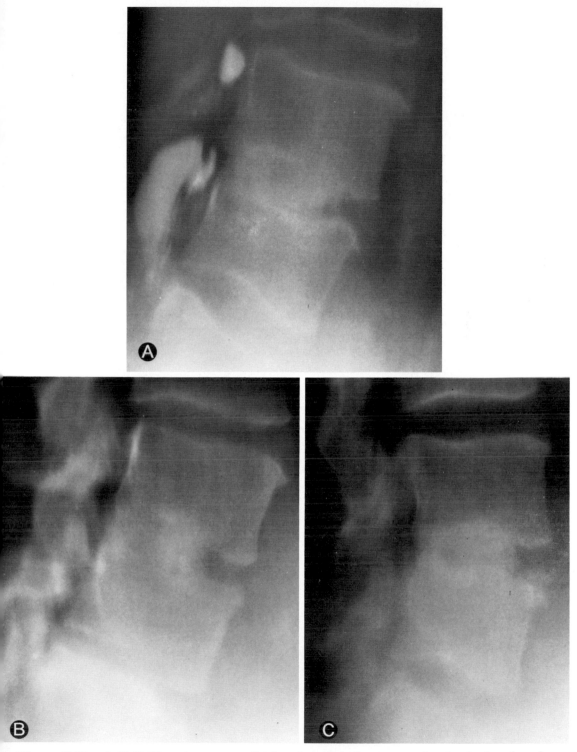

Figure 7.29. A, B, C. Three tomograms all taken 4 months after surgery show beginning of good osteosynthesis.

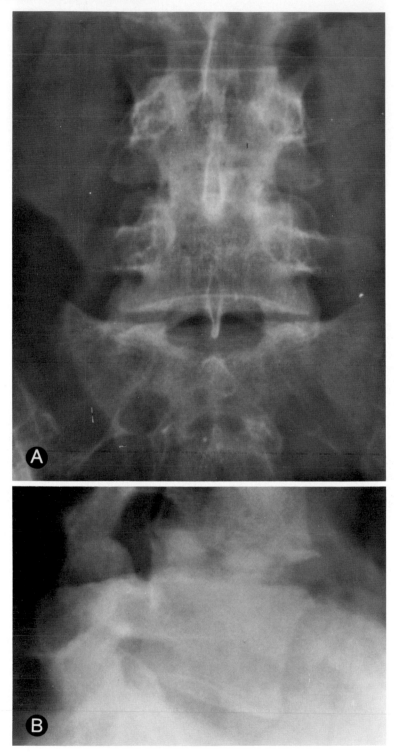

Figure 7.30. A and B. AP and lateral. Two years postoperative. Plain AP and lateral lumbar spine x-rays show solid bony fusion in the disc space with evidence of trabeculation.

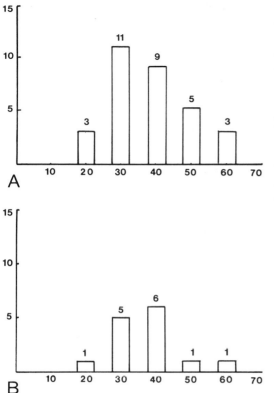

A

B

Figure 7.31. At 2 years of follow-up, 45 patients are shown by age and sex distribution (A. male, B. female).

questionable fusion; all of the rest had solid fusion (Fig. 7.33A). In the good group, three had fusion and three did not have fusion. In those three cases of nonunion, motion was detected but the disc space was not collapsed indicating the possibility that incomplete bony union still may be followed by good results. Fourteen patients were in the unsatisfactory group, which included 10 patients with secondary gain problems and all but one of these patients had radiologic evidence of fusion. It seems that in the secondary gain group, the status of the fusion does not correlate with clinical result (Fig. 7.33B).

In the unsatisfactory group, four patients had no secondary gain and three had evidence of motion of pseudoarthrosis. Excluding patients in the secondary gain category,

solid bony fusion seems to be a prerequisite for an excellent result.

Of the 45 patients, 34 (75%) returned to work (Fig. 7.35). Nine kept their previous heavy duty jobs and seven had to be downgraded to lighter duty work, even though they still performed physical manual occupations. If we remove the patients with secondary gain from this group, 33 patients (97%) returned to work after surgery. Sixteen patients of this group had previous disc surgery at the same level (Fig. 7.36). In this category, eight had excellent result (50%) and one had good result (6%) giving a total of 56% satisfactory result. Excluding the patients with secondary gain (6) from this series, then 70% had excellent result and 10% had good result, thus giving a total of 80% with satisfactory result.

DISCUSSION

Froning and Frohman[19] demonstrated limitation of flexion extension movement in the majority of patients with successful discectomy. Persistent mobility, comparable to that expected in a normal individual, usually was found in patients judged to have had a poor result. This supports the contention of posterior interbody fusion advocates that to achieve a better result in disc prolapse surgery, there should be minimal movement of the motion segment after surgery.

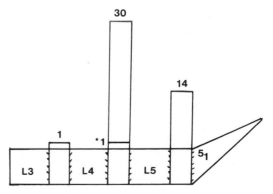

Figure 7.32. Distribution of surgery at level of disc spaces. * Two-level fusion L3–4 and L4–5.

A. CLINICAL RESULT OF ALL PATIENTS (45)

	EXCELLENT	GOOD	FAIR	POOR
45 PATIENTS	25 (55.5%)	6 (13.3%)	7 (15.5%)	7 (15.5%)

SATISFACTORY RESULT 68.8%   UNSATISFACTORY RESULT 31.2%

B. CLINICAL RESULT EXCLUDING PATIENTS WITH SECONDARY GAIN

	EXCELLENT	GOOD	FAIR	POOR
35 PATIENTS	24 (70.6%)	6 (17.6%)	3 (8.7%)	1 (3.1%)

SATISFACTORY GROUP 88.2%   UNSATISFACTORY GROUP 11.8%

Figure 7.33. A. 82% fusion in 45 patients with 2 years of follow-up correlate with results. B. Fusion rate and result in 11 patients with secondary gain problems at 2 years of follow-up.

Simeone, in discussing a paper[10] stated that

"the issue of indication for lumbar fusion remains unsettled. Classically, the neurosurgeons frequently have referred lumbar fusion procedures to their orthopaedic colleagues. Independent of one's feelings about fusion, the surgeon who believes in lumbar fusion should be familiar with this approach ... On logical grounds, one must assume that the posterior interbody fusion approach is at least equal to the more formidable transabdominal anterior lumbar fusion, during which the nerve roots can be less adequately inspected ... Spine surgeons who believe in fusion should have this procedure in their technical repertoire."

Burton and Finneson,[14] reviewing their combined experience with failed back surgery syndrome (FBSS), found that 50–60% had evidence of lateral spinal stenosis at the time of their first lumbar discectomy. The clinical importance of lateral spinal stenosis as a clinical entity, with or without disc herniation, only recently has been fully appreciated. We must consider posterior lumbar interbody fusion as an ideal definitive reconstructive and curative procedure for lateral spinal stenosis with concomitant subarticular nerve entrapment (Figs. 7.4–7.6). When the compressed pair of nerves are effectively decompressed at the lateral recesses and at the foramen, there is a loss of stability unless the altered dynamic motion segment dysfunction is stabilized by fusion. Without this, facet hypertrophy and tropism would surely recur. The cause of tropism and hypertrophy of the posterior joints or facets are best explained by Wolff's law which states that "any changes of bony architecture are the result of external environment."[15] Failure to eliminate the effects of lateral spinal stenosis and to prevent its recurrence is one of the most important causes of failure of relief by a simple lumbar discectomy, leading to repeated similar procedures and FBSS. We too often blame the failure on the lack of motivation of the patient. We must consider that, in many cases, FBSS is due to a failure of operative technique.

Modern improvements in operative illumination, better control of epidural hemorrhage by proper positioning of the patient, and the use of Surgicel as a tampon in retracting epidural veins and dura definitely improve the technical feasibility of PLIF. Adherence to Cloward's teaching, which emphasizes impacting the disc space with as many bone grafts as possible, and including cancellous bone to fill all available spaces, which would likely be followed by a higher rate of spinal fusion, would improve the outcome of PLIF procedures.

McNab[16] in his text, *Backache* stated that a solitary bone graft in the disc space would be absorbed by the surrounding fibrous tissue. He advised[17] that " . . . to have a successful interbody fusion, then the only substance between the vertebral bodies must be bone." Bunnell's[18] experimental work with anterior interbody fusion on canines also indicates that only those spaces packed tightly with graft material were likely to produce fusion in his series. His work favors cancellous bone on cortical bone as the ideal graft material in interbody fusion.

In surgery on recurrent disc problems, it is wise not to adhere to the surgical principle that the dura and nerve root be visual-

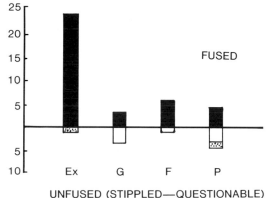

A. 45 PATIENTS WITH 2-YEAR FOLLOW-UP

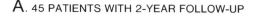

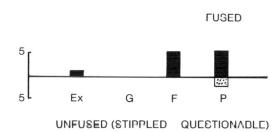

B. 11 PATIENTS WITH SECONDARY GAIN

Figure 7.34. A. Clinical result of patients. B. Clinical result with secondary pain problems.

A
9 Holding heavy duty
7 Downgraded to lighter duty
34/45 = 75%

B
Without secondary gain problem
33/34 = 97%

Figure 7.35. A. Percentage of return to work—75%. B. Percentage of return to work without secondary gain problems—97%.

CLINICAL RESULT OF POSTERIOR
LUMBAR INTERBODY FUSION IN
POST-DISCECTOMY PATIENTS

Combined (16)		Without Secondary Gain (10)	
Excellent	Good	Excellent	Good
8 (50%)	1 (6%)	7 (56%)	1 (10%)
Satisfactory 56%		Satisfactory 70%	

Figure 7.36. Clinical result in patients who had previous lumbar discectomies.

ized before retracting and exposing the disc space. Where there is scar tissue, it would be wise to remove the medial one-half of the facet and gain entrance to the lateral gutter, lateral to the nerve root. Once the disc space is entered, the scar tissue around the nerve root easily can be identified and pushed medially.

In cases of spondylolisthesis, posterior lumbar interbody fusion for slippage beyond Grade I is technically difficult, but not impossible. In our series, we only removed the posterior 75–85% of the disc for fear of endangering the great vessels in front of the vertebral disc. Anterior remnants of disc material are allowed to remain attached to the anterior longitudinal ligament. We further believe that, in posterior lumbar interbody fusion, there should be more than 50% of the disc space filled with bone grafts. Since it is difficult to reduce the slippage in spondylolisthesis, even in the most ideal cases of Grade I, only about 50% of exposed and opposing surfaces of the intervertebral surfaces can receive bone grafts. Therefore, with any slippage beyond Grade I, we would recommend posterior lateral fusion.

CONCLUSION

(1) Posterior lumbar interbody fusion not only has the advantage of avoiding collapse of the disc space, it assures stability of the motion segment. The stability would avoid tropism of the facet, frequently a cause of recurrent lateral spinal stenosis and FBSS. It also accomplishes wide decompression of all neural components and distraction of the intervertebral disc space. The natural posterior concavity of the lumbar spine produces a firm locking mechanism of the grafts within the disc space. With a generous number of bone grafts, both cortical peg grafts and cancellous grafts, tightly impacted into the disc space, solid fusion is enhanced.

(2) The modified technique[10] of posterior lumbar interbody fusion with preservation of the facet spinous processes, supraspinous ligaments, and cortical plate alleviates the postoperative slippage and settlement. The integrity of involved motion segment is scrupulously maintained.

(3) Forty-five cases who had undergone modified posterior lumbar interbody fusion with at least 2 years of follow-up show 82% bony fusion as visualized by radiologic technique, with clinical result rated as satisfactory in 68.8%. Patients who had previous disc surgery done at the same level had a satisfactory result of 56%. Eleven patients who had secondary gain problems were removed from consideration. The overall satisfactory result would be 88.2% and, in patients who had previous disc surgery done at the same level, the satisfactory result would be 80%.

(4) Experience with over 300 PLIF cases indicates that the posterior lumbar interbody fusion should be utilized more widely as a reconstructive procedure for disabling lumbar degenerative disc disease.

References

1. Cloward, R. B.: The treatment of ruptured lumbar intervertebral discs by vertebral body fusion. Indications, operative technique, after care. *J. Neurosurg. 10*:154–168, 1953.
2. Cloward, R. B.: New treatment of ruptured intervertebral disc. Read at the annual meeting of the Hawaii Territorial Medical Association, May 1945.
3. Cloward, R. B.: Lesions of intervertebral discs and their treatment by intervertebral fusion method. *Clin. Orthop. 27*:51–77, 1963.
4. Crock, H. V.: Isolated lumbar disc resorption as a cause of nerve root canal stenosis. *Clin. Orthop. 191*:109–115, 1976.
5. LeVay, D.: A survey of surgical management of lumbar disc prolapse in the United Kingdom and Eire. *Lancet 1*:1211–1213, 1967.
6. Junghanns, J., Schmorl, G.: *The Human Spine in Health and Disease.* Second edition. New York, N.Y., Grune & Stratton, 1971, p. 35–37.
7. Wiltberger, B. R.: The prefit dowel intervertebral body fusion as used in lumbar disc therapy. A preliminary report. *Am. J. Surg. 6*:723–727, 1953.
8. Wiltberger, B. R.: Intervertebral body fusion by the use of posterior bone dowel. *Clin. Orthop. 35*:69–79, 1964.
9. Keim, H. A.: Indication for spinal fusion and techniques. *Clin. Neurosurg. 25*:266–267, 1977.
10. Lin, P. M.: A technical modification of Cloward's posterior lumbar interbody fusion. *Neurosurgery 1(2)*:124, 1977.
11. Robinson, R. A.: Anterior and posterior cervical spine fusion. *Clin. Orthop. 35*:34–62, 1964.

12. Robinson, R. A., Smith, G. W.: Anterolateral cervical disc removal and interbody fusion for cervical disc syndrome. *Bull. Johns Hopk. Hosp. 96:*223–224, 1955.
13. Froning, E. C., Frohman, B.: Motion of the lumbosacral spine after laminectomy and spine fusion. Correlation of motion with the result. *J. Bone Joint Surg. 50:*897–918, 1968.
14. Burton, C., Finneson, B.: Failed Back Surgery. Presented at the Lumbar Spine Surgery Seminar, Gainesville, FL, 1980.
15. Wolf's Law, Dorlands Medical Dictionary, 25th Edition, W. B. Saunders, Philadelphia, PA, 1974, p. 843.
16. McNab, I.: Chapter 2. In *Backache.* Baltimore, MD, Williams & Wilkins, 1977, p. 166.
17. McNab, I. Personal communication, December 1979.
18. Bunnell, W. P.: Anterior spinal fusion: Promising canine data. Presented at Eastern Orthopedic Association as an award paper for spinal research. Miami, FL, October 17–21, 1979.

8

The Place of Spinal Fusion in Lumbar Intervertebral Joint Disease

In this chapter, I will discuss the place of spinal fusion in the treatment of lumbar intervertebral joint disease. This, of course, includes intervertebral disc disease. Herein lies the real controversy as to the place of fusion. Few would question its efficacy in such conditions as spondylolisthesis in children or fracture dislocation of the lumbar spine, especially when used in conjunction with some metallic internal fixation in scoliosis or spinal tuberculosis.[1, 2]

Since the beginning of disc surgery, lumbar fusion has been inextricably bound to discectomy. December 31, 1932 was the first time that a disc fragment was removed when it was recognized as such and not thought to be a chrondroma. A fusion was done in conjunction.[3, 4] It seemed so very logical to do a fusion after disc removal. If the annulus is incised and the nucleus pulposus removed, then surely an unstable segment must be produced and fusion should be added—so the reasoning went. At that time, fusion was nearly always done from L4 to S1. It seemed illogical to do a so-called "floating fusion" (in other words, not to extend the fusion to the sacrum). As one doctor put it,[5] "just move the sacrum up a couple of notches." Since we so seldom see trouble from nerve root pressure down in the sacrum, if one could extend the sacrum up a few segments, theoretically, one could bypass the area where most of the trouble occurs.

Caldwell and Sheppard,[6] in a classic article in 1948 entitled "Criteria for spine fusion following removal of a protruded nucleus pulposus," said, "excellent and satisfactory results can be obtained in as high a percentage of cases by laminectomy alone as by the combined operation." They concluded that "there are no criteria for spine fusion following removal of a protruded nucleus pulposus."

Most recent reports of the good or excellent results following laminectomy and discectomy have been in the neighborhood of 70%.[7] If a fusion has been added, then success rate goes up by a relatively few percentage points, perhaps 70–75%. However, invariably, the author hastens to add that the difference is not statistically significant. Why this small difference?[8] Perhaps it is because the two operations are done for different reasons. A discectomy is done for pressure on the neural elements and a fusion is done for instability. It is likely that a discectomy done through a small hemilaminectomy does not produce instability of a sufficient degree that the percentage of good results would be increased by adding a fusion. Thus, in this situation, adding a fusion is unnecessary and so does not significantly increase the percentage of good results. There are times, however, when a fusion is beneficial and this accounts for the small improvement in results by adding a fusion. Just what the circumstances are which make adding a fusion beneficial have yet to be clearly delineated.

From the time I opened my office for the practice of orthopaedic surgery early in 1946 until about 1968, our policy (unless there was some definite condition such as spondylolisthesis or disc resorption) was to do a discectomy through one or two hemilaminectomies but not to fuse. About one case in ten either suffered a recurrence of disc herniation or was sufficiently unrelieved to require a second operation. This second operation consisted of a fusion and laminectomy or, possibly, a fusion alone. On this second surgery, our good or excellent clinical results were 60–65%.

The implication is that, in most cases of disc herniation, the cause of pain is nerve root pressure and that whatever herniation is present without nerve pressure is not likely to produce pain.

At the present state of the art, there are relatively few things that can be done surgically for a bulging herniated disc. One can remove the pressure from the neural elements by removing the bulging portion of the disc or by removing the bone over the disc. Pressure may also be removed by injecting the disc with chymopapain or collagenase. The other way is to remove the motion of one or more segments with a fusion. If a fusion is contemplated, the herniated disc is usually removed before fusion.

A most interesting phenomenon noted in the literature is that in several large stud-

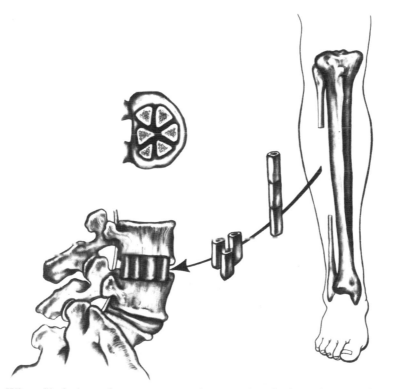

Figure 8.1. When fibula is used, use great care in removing the bone from the leg so as not to injure the superficial peroneal nerve as it lies very close to the anterior surface of the fibula in its upper third. Use Henry's approach. Use small dissectors such as ligamentum flavum dissectors to separate the periosteum from the fibular bone. Do not use large retractors such as Bennets as these may stretch the nerve. Go no lower than the mid- and lower thirds and do not divide the interosseus membrane below that level as it will make the ankle unstable. Reprinted with permission from AAOS Instructional Course. St. Louis, MO, C. V. Mosby, 1979.

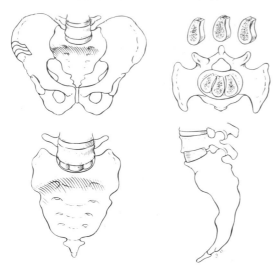

Figure 8.2. Horse-shoe grafts are taken from the crest of the ilium near the thickest portion anteriorly. Three or four of these are put in. After the space seems to be totally full, two slightly curved Lambotte osteotomes can be put in and the grafts levered laterally and thus room made for yet another graft. Reprinted from Ruge, D., Wiltse, L. L.: Spondylolisthesis and its treatment; conservative treatment, fusion with and without reduction. In *Spinal Disorders: Diagnosis and Treatment.* Philadelphia, Lea & Febiger, 1977.

ies[8, 9] of spinal fusion done in conjunction with discectomy, those who developed a pseudoarthrosis after attempted fusion did as well clinically as matched cases who obtained a solid fusion.[10] Taken at its face value, this would indicate that the fusion operation is valueless. The probable explanation is that the fusion was not indicated in the first place. In all likelihood, a discectomy alone would have done as well. As of this writing, I seldom do a fusion in conjunction with a simple discectomy when this is the primary operation. I will say, however, that I am swinging back to doing more fusions than in the previous 10–15 years.

FUSION IN SPINAL STENOSIS

The major problem in the surgical treatment of spinal stenosis is how to decom-

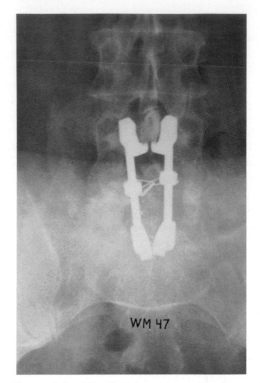

Figure 8.3. Knodt rods are occasionally used either for compression or distraction. Here we can see them used for distraction. In this situation, they serve a function for stability, however. I prefer them for compression. Reprinted from Wiltse, L. L.: Surgery for intervertebral disc disease of the lumbar spine. *Clin. Orthop. 129:*33, 1977.

press adequately and still preserve stability. Back stability and decompression are important.

The advent of computerized axial tomography (CAT) has added a whole new dimension to our diagnostic ability in regard to the location of compression in spinal stenosis. Compression can take place at any of the following points.

(A) Central canal stenosis
    (1) Disc (central), soft or calcified
    (2) Osteophytes at rim of vertebral bodies
    (3) Congenital stenosis of either central or lateral canals
    (4) Hard bulging annulus
(B) Lateral entrapment

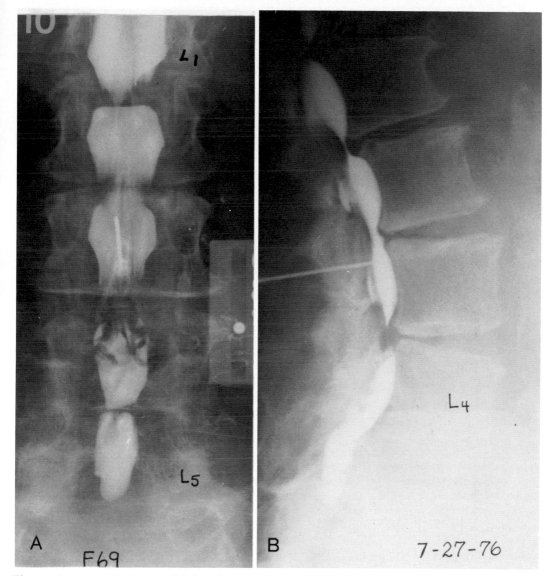

Figure 8.4. A. A 66-year-old female with very severe multilevel stenosis and early partial paralysis about both hips is shown. The level with the most severe stenosis was L1. B. The only reason to fuse in such a case is at levels where it is necessary to totally unstabilize posteriorly. I would not attempt a long multilevel fusion after a long decompression. Reprinted from AAOS Instructional Course. St. Louis, MO, C. V. Mosby Co., 1979.

(1) Between medial swing of superior articular process and bulging annulus or osteophytic lower rim of body of vertebra above

(2) Anywhere from this point out to the lateral end of the foramen due to:

(a) lateral disc protrusion, either soft or hard
(b) the ala of the sacrum
(c) osteophytic rim of the bodies of the vertebrae

(3) Between the caudal edge of the pedicle and a hard rolled up an-

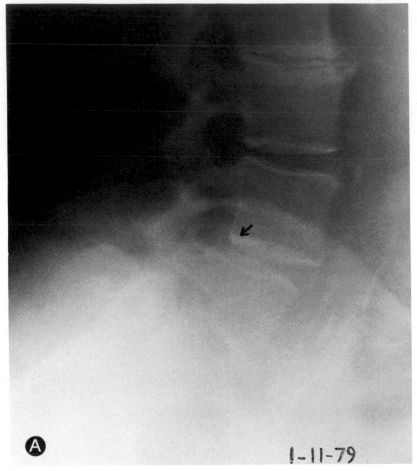

1-11-79

Figure 8.5. A 66-year-old female with spinal stenosis is shown. A total decompression of all posterior elements had been done in a distant city. The Preoperative lateral (A), preoperative AP myelogram (B), preoperative lateral myelogram (C) are shown. D. Shows a drawing of type of decompression done. (Reprinted from AAOS Instructional Course. St. Louis, MO, C. V. Mosby Co., 1979.) I believe this was an unnecessarily radical decompression. E. Shows the x-ray of decompression. F. Within a few months postdecompression, this type of collapse had occurred and the patient had fairly marked weakness of muscles supplied by L3, L4, and L5 spinal nerves, more severe on the left. G. Harrington rods were placed from the ala of the sacrum to T11 and good reduction obtained. At this time, a transverse process fusion was done from L3 to L5. Two weeks later, an anterior interbody fusion was done, keying a large slab of iliac crest into the bodies. She was kept flat for 2 more months, then allowed up in a body jacket. At this writing, she is markedly improved and her paralysis is gone. The fusion appears to be solid.

nulus or even the superior border of the body of the vertebra below in spondylolisthesis

(4) Between the transverse process and (we have dubbed this the "far out" syndrome):

(a) a bulging annulus

(b) the ala of the sacrum

(c) an osteoarthritic rim of bodies of the vertebra

(d) a combination of the above

A CAT scan can show these areas and a skillful radiologist can estimate the degree of compression.

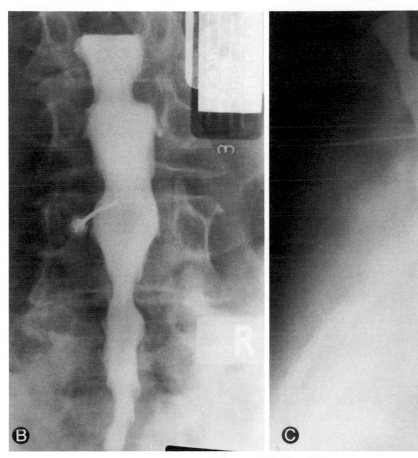

Figure 8.5. B and C.

How then can we adequately decompress far laterally and still preserve stability? Six possible answers are as follows:

(1) If the disc space is very narrow and osteoarthritic, there may be enough stability enabling us to totally remove all posterior support. Fortunately, the most severe cases of stenosis often have narrowed osteoarthritic disc spaces.

(2) Do a Cloward-type[18] posterior interbody fusion totally decompressing and fusing. The problem has arisen that when all support from the posterior elements is removed, failure of fusion may be present in an unacceptably high percentage of cases.

(3) Do an anterior interbody fusion, using fibula as a grafting material, jacking the vertebrae apart very severely. Fibular bone is so hard that it will not settle. Distraction lifts the bodies apart and takes pressure off the nerves in the lateral canals. We have found this to work rather well. Once a fusion is solid, a posterior, total decompression can be done if necessary (Fig. 8.1).

(4) Do an anterior interbody fusion using ilium. This graft is softer and we must depend on the removal of motion combined with some lifting of the vertebral bodies to relieve the pain. Figure 8.2 shows this type of fusion.

(5) Perform a posterolateral fusion combined with rods of some type to jack the vertebral bodies apart. Figure 8.3 demonstrates this.

(6) Do a simple posterior fusion and depend on the eventual rigidity to relieve the pain. This is not as farfetched as it may seem. This may be why we obtained as

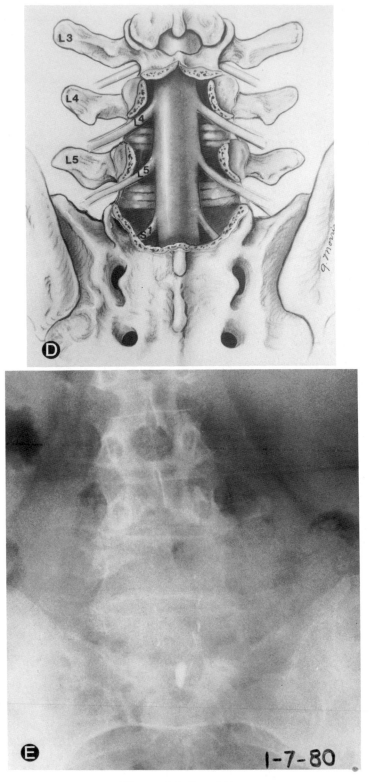

Figure 8.5. D and E.

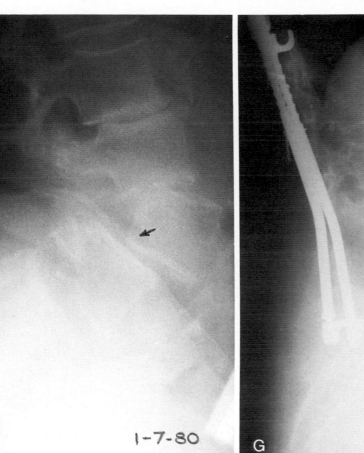

F 1-7-80

G 18 MAR 80

Figure 8.5. F and G.

many good results as we did in the years 1946–1968 when our routine was to do discectomies first and, later, to perform fusion in those patients who failed to get relief.

The problem is that many cases of spinal stenosis involve several levels. When there are as many levels to be decompressed as we see in Figure 8.4A and B, it would seem that fusion would be impractical. We are seeing this type of problem frequently now.

Rosomoff[11] has done total posterior element removal of a large series of patients who had had several previous surgeries. He reports that he has not had much trouble with instability. However, in my experience, olisthesis or collapse of the spine has occurred often enough after total posterior element removal that I save the pars interarticularis and lateral masses unless the disc spaces are very narrow.

Figure 8.5A–G shows a 66-year-old woman who had a total decompression done for spinal stenosis in April, 1979. It should be noted that the disc spaces are fairly normal in width. After the decompression, her spine started to collapse and she began to show signs of nerve compression. She lost dorsiflexion power in her left foot and experienced considerable weakness in the left quadriceps. Because of progressive nerve paralysis and collapse, it was believed that reduction and stabilization was necessary.

First, Harrington rods were placed posteriorly from the alae of the sacrum to the lamina of T11, lengthening the lumbar spine and bringing about good correction. In the same operation, a transverse process fusion was done from L3 to L5. A fusion was not done from L5 to the sacrum be-

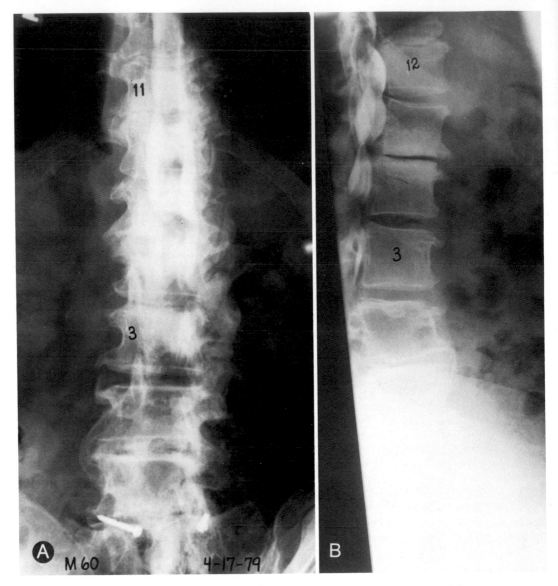

Figure 8.6. This 60-year-old male had severe symptoms of spinal stenosis. There was a near total block at L2 and several other levels were nearly blocked. He had a marked motor weakness of several levels but especially in the muscles supplied by the L2 spinal nerve on the left. AP myelogram before operation is shown (A). Note very little metrizamide can be seen because of the severe stenosis. The lateral myelogram before operation is shown (B). Note the near block at the L2 level. C. Shows the long decompression done. Pars were all saved but at L2 they could not be saved. The disc space at L2 is seen to be fairly wide which is dangerous to stability. D. Shows the lateral view 9 months after operation. At the level of total decompression, olisthesis is developing. The patient had done well clinically. E. Because it was feared that olisthesis would continue, an anterior interbody fusion was done at L2 using fibular struts. As of this writing, he is doing well clinically and the graft seems to be nearly incorporated.

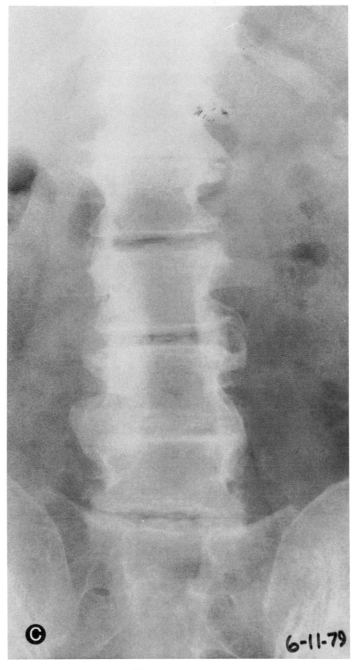

Figure 8.6. C.

cause this level was not unstable and showed no change in position. It was believed that arthrodesis probably would not occur without an added anterior interbody fusion since we would not expect bone to jump from one transverse process to another, the lateral masses having been removed. Approximately 2.5 weeks after the posterior operation, an anterior interbody fusion was done from L3 to L5, using a large

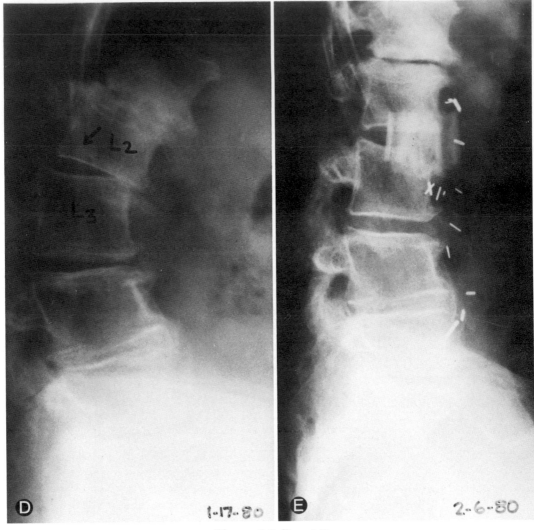

Figure 8.6. D and E.

slab of iliac crest keyed into the vertebral bodies. The patient was kept in a horizontal position for approximately 8 weeks and then allowed up in a plastic brace. As of this writing, she has recovered from her rather severe paralysis of the left leg and the fusion is solid.

If the disc spaces are very narrow and osteoarthritic, the danger of instability is less. However, it is difficult to be sure just how much narrowing need be present to be reasonably sure collapse will not occur (Fig. 8.6A and B). This series of x-rays shows a 60-year-old male who came in because of increasing paralysis in the lower extremities plus very severe pain and difficulty in walking. He was first seen in February, but because he was an accountant and his business depended on his being in the office, he had to wait until after April 15. Before April 15 arrived, paralysis had progressed. A CAT scan was done which showed he had very severe spinal stenosis far up the spine, even at the T12 level. However at the L2 level, the block was near total and the compression reached clear out through the lateral canals compressing the spinal nerves all the way out to the base of the transverse proc-

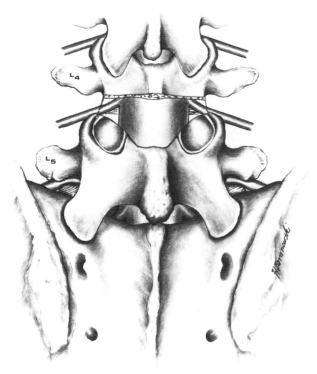

Figure 8.7. This drawing shows a type of decompression which has some danger. If much olisthesis develops after operation with this narrow decompression, the cauda equina will be compressed and paralysis may result. A longer decompression is safer if it must be total.

esses. He had a "far out" syndrome at this L2 level.

A decompression was done as shown in Figure 8.6C. Because of the total block at L2, it was necessary to remove all posterior support including the articular processes and bases of the transverse processes at that level.

He made a rather dramatic symptomatic recovery after the operation and resumed his accounting work in a matter of days. He sat in his hospital bed working. Everything seemed to be going well until x-rays were taken 6–8 months after surgery (Fig. 8.6D). It was noted that there was anterior displacement of L2 on L3 where total decompression had been done even though we had thought the disc space was narrow enough that olisthesis would not occur. Because this is rather high in the lumbar spine and the lower end of the spinal cord is here, we believed that stabilization was mandatory. Since all the elements had been re-

moved posteriorly, it would be difficult to do a posterior fusion. Therefore, an anterior interbody fusion was chosen. This was done with fibular graft (Fig. 8.6E). (If fibular graft is used, the segments of graft must be stood on end and the vertebral bodies blocked apart very severely.) He was having very little pain before the operation and the operation was done prophylactically. He did well postoperatively and, as of this writing, is doing well. The fusion is now solid.

The question naturally arises—how dangerous is it for anterior slip to occur? It seems that a moderate amount of slip or even a severe amount sometimes is not dangerous, providing that a long decompression has been done posteriorly. If, however, a short decompression has been done posteriorly and significant slip occurs, it can produce paraplegia as was seen in one case. Figure 8.7 shows a drawing of a case we saw in conference where a short

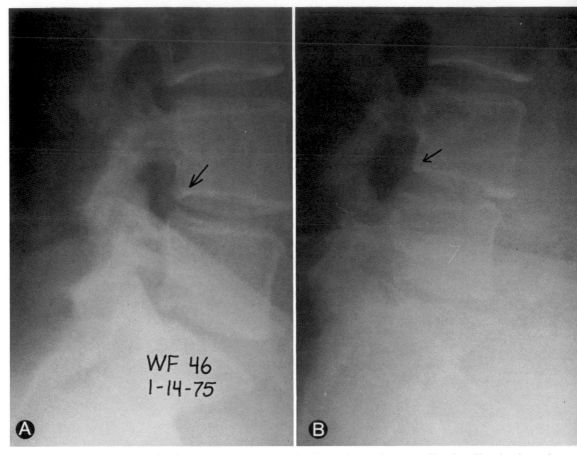

WF 46
1-14-75

Figure 8.8. Knutsen's phenomenon is shown. A. Note that, when standing bending backwards, there is nearly normal alignment. B. When the patient is bending forward in a sitting position on a very low stool shows abnormal tilt and anterior translation of L4 on L5 is shown.

decompression was done removing all the posterior support including the articular processes. In addition, the disc was entered. Olisthesis occurred and, because the decompression was so short, the cauda equina was, in effect, in a shears and the patient became paraplegic.

Solid fusion in the lumbar spine can be fairly hard to accomplish. Sometimes it may be necessary to fuse both anteriorly and posteriorly. If this is the course decided upon, it probably is well to do the posterior fusion first. Then, after 10–12 days, do the anterior fusion. Whether to let the patient up immediately or keep him in a horizontal position for several weeks depends on the

stability of the fusion. Most of the time, we let our patients up immediately, but if there is severe instability and the graft is none too secure (especially the anterior graft), it is wise to keep them lying down for 6–8 weeks.

If instability is what makes fusion necessary, the question naturally arises—how much instability must be present to warrant a fusion? Figure 8.8A and B shows a rather common situation. Here is a woman in her 40's whose x-ray looks rather normal when she is in a standing position but on flexion, we see the typical anterior translation of L4 on L5. This is often the precursor of degenerative spondylolisthesis. In a middle-aged female, if we wait 5–10 years after the appearance of this kind of instability, we often find on x-ray that the patient has developed degenerative spondylolisthesis. If this patient is having a great deal of pain, we certainly could consider an L4 to L5 fusion. However, the fact is that a very large number of patients will show this phenomenon and have no pain. Mensor and Duvall[12] have shown that middle-aged women with this phenomenon have low back pain twice as often as those without. However, it is still in the neighborhood of 8–16%. As a result, fusion is seldom done for this type of instability seen on x-ray.

Figure 8.9A–D shows the x-rays, myelogram, and a drawing of a patient with very severe spinal stenosis. A total decompression and no olisthesis occurred. It is safe to do a total decompression where there is marked stability by osteoarthritis and disc space narrowing. No spinal fusion is necessary, but this disc space narrowing must be severe.

There is another theoretical consideration to be taken into account. It is our belief that a solid anterior interbody fusion is adequate in the cervical spine. The osteophytes tend to disappear and space is gained for the cord which lies posteriorly. Motion is stopped and a certain amount of neurologic recovery takes place. Likewise, in the young teenager with high-grade slip in spondylolisthesis (even though the patient has foot drop, reflex change, and marked sensory change with tight hamstrings), if a solid posterior fusion can be obtained, even though no decompression is done, nearly all regain muscle strength and lose their numbness and tight hamstrings. Thus, in these situations, neurologic change has tended to disappear by nothing more than removing motion. What actually happens to reverse the neurologic change? In spondylolisthesis, does the pulsation of the subarachnoid space cause a little increase in size of the passageway for the nerves at the L5-S1 level? Or did the spinal nerves accommodate to the cramped quarters? No one has explained this point. We know that in animal experiments, when compression is gradual, nerves can actually be compressed to one-fourth of their size and still function normally.

By the same reasoning then, in the 60-year-old patient with high-grade spinal stenosis from T12 down and with multiple levels markedly stenosed (Fig. 8.6), if we could get a solid fusion from T12 to S1, would not the symptoms of spinal stenosis be relieved? It should not be impossible to achieve a fusion using Harrington rods and a large amount of bone posterolaterally. The fact is, that for unknown reasons, solid fusion does not seem to reverse the process in the adult lumbar spine as it does in the cervical spine. Decompression seems to be necessary in the lumbar spine of the older person.

INDICATIONS AND TECHNIQUES FOR SPINAL FUSION

Degenerative Spondylolisthesis

If fusion is indicated for instability, certainly degenerative spondylolisthesis at L4 is the classic situation. Therefore, spinal fusion would seem, at least on a theoretical basis, to be indicated. Figure 8.10A–I shows a series of pictures of a case of degenerative spondylolisthesis. It has been our practice, in people under the physiologic age of 65 years, to add a fusion between L4 and L5 only. As long as the lateral masses are saved and the facets are not interfered with, fusion at this one level occurs without much difficulty.

However, the question still arises—is fusion really necessary in the first place? The difference in the subjective clinical end result in a group whom we fused and a matched group whom we did not fuse was not statistically significant.[7] In spite of our own statistics, we still perform fusion on patients below age 70 if instability is severe

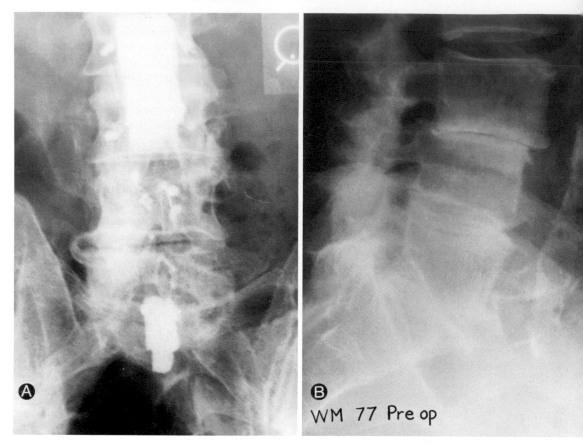

WM 77 Pre op

Figure 8.9.   This case of a 77-year-old male illustrates the principle that, if the disc spaces are very narrow, there is sufficient stability so that olisthesis will not occur and a fusion is not necessary. A. Preoperative AP myelogram is shown. Note the severe block. B. Lateral view shows marked narrowing of the disc spaces at the three lowest levels. (Reprinted from AAOS Instructional Course, St. Louis, MO, C. V. Mosby Co., 1979.) C. A very nearly total posterior decompression was done as shown in this x-ray. D. A drawing of total decompression, 3-level, is shown. Use this severe amount of decompression only if very severe osteoarthritis is present as seen here. When last seen 2 years postoperation, the patient was free of pain. The x-ray showed no further olisthesis at any level. L3 showed the same dgree of slip as before operation.

(as it usually is). But the rather marked success of decompression, whether or not fusion is added, again would tend to fortify the proposition that decompression of the neural elements is what counts and that stability is a secondary consideration.

Midline Approach for Spinal Fusion

We have used this approach relatively infrequently (Fig. 8.11A and B) in the last 20 years. When we do use it, it is usually in conjunction with a midline decompression in cases of degenerative spondylolisthesis. We virtually never lay bone graft over exposed nerves as bone tends to grow around the nerves and cause pain.

The Paraspinal Sacrospinalis-Splitting Approach to the Lumbar Spine

The paraspinal approach[13] to the lumbar spine passes trans-sacrospinalis. The sacrospinalis muscle is split about two fingerbreadths lateral to the midline (Fig. 8.12A–D). The transverse processes and lateral

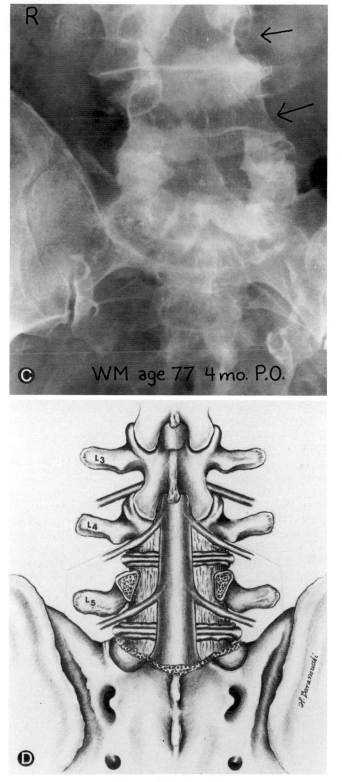

Figure 8.9. C and D.

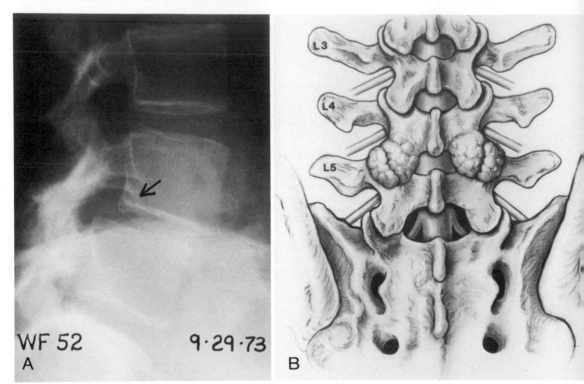

Figure 8.10. Here is a case of degenerative spondylolisthesis in a 52-year-old woman. A. The lateral view preoperation is shown. Note degree of slip. Compare degree of slip with final lateral and note mild increase. This is common. B. This is a drawing of typical degenerative spondylolisthesis at L4. C. Note the typical hourglass constriction on myelogram. (Reprinted from AAOS Instructional Course. St. Louis, MO, C. V. Mosby & Co., 1979.) D. This is the type of decompression done in most cases but not in this case. E. A small decompression which can be done and was done in this particular case. We wonder if saving a sliver of lamina is of any benefit. F. This is a cross-section of decompression. Note it is the inferior articular processes of L4 which compress the L5 spinal nerves. (Reprinted from Wiltse, L. L.: Surgery for intervertebral disc disease of the lumbar spine. *Clin. Orthop. 129:* 33–39, 1977.) G. A drawing of the type of fusion done in this case is shown. (Reprinted from Wiltse, L. L.: Common problems of the lumbar spine: degenerative spondylolisthesis and spinal stenosis. *J. Con. Educ. Orthop.* May, 1979.) H. An AP x-ray of fusion is shown. I. A lateral x-ray of fusion is shown. Note some increase in slip. (Reprinted from AAOS Instructional Course. St. Louis, MO, C. V. Mosby & Co., 1979.)

masses are reached more directly through this approach and there is no more bleeding than from a midline approach to the lateral parts of the vertebrae.

Operative Technique

The patient is placed on the operating table in the kneeling position. A midline skin incision is made but, once through the skin, the skin is retracted so the fascial incision can be made two fingerbreadths lateral to the spinous processes and three-quarters of the way out laterally on the sacrospinalis. These fascial incisions can be curved slightly toward the midline at their caudal ends.

Cutting the fascia transversely for this short distance allows better retraction. Above the level of L5, the lumbosacral muscle mass separates rather easily into two muscle groups—the multifidus medially and the iliocostalis lumborum laterally. The

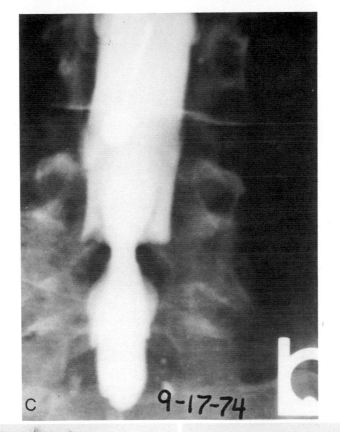

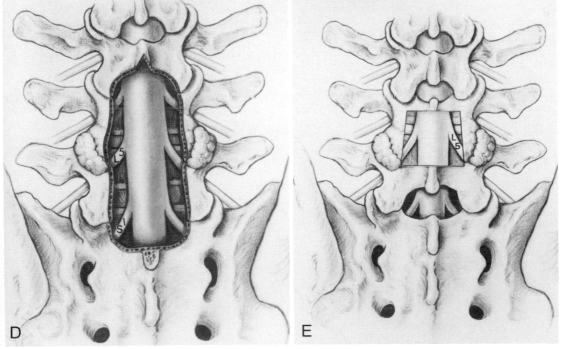

Figure 8.10. C, D, and E.

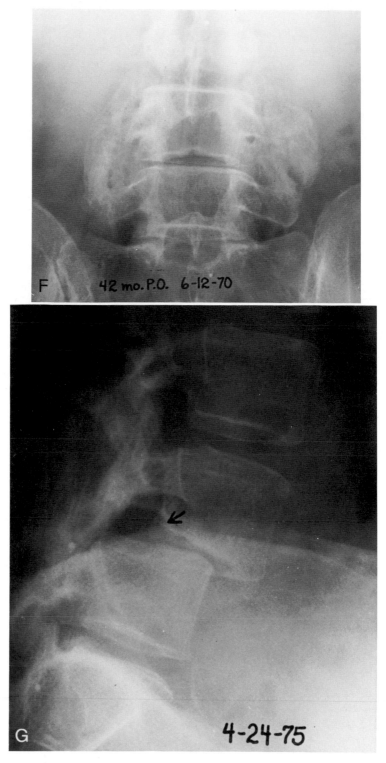

Figure 8.10. F and G.

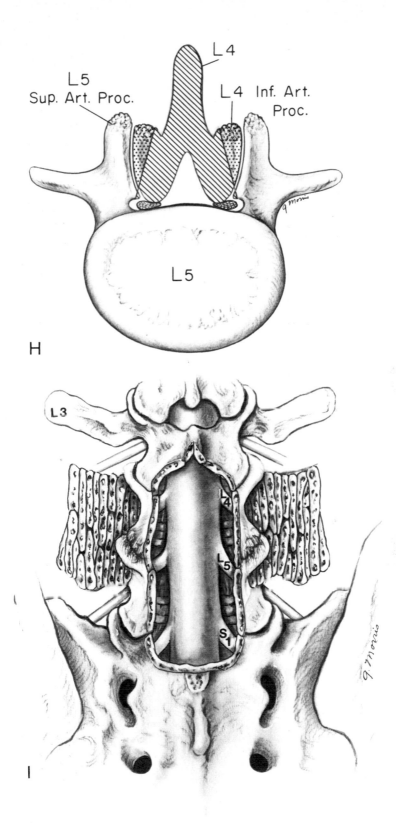

L4

L5
Sup. Art. Proc.

L4 Inf. Art.
Proc.

L5

H

L3

L4

L5

S1

I

Figure 8.10. H and I.

147

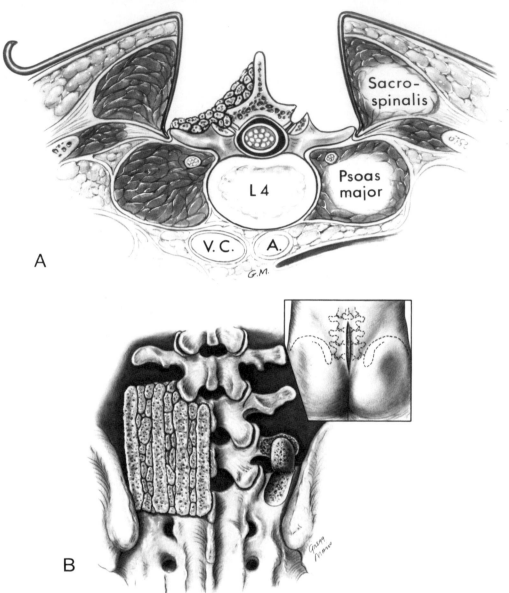

Figure 8.11. Midline approach for lumbar spinal fusion. A. The skin incision is midline and all tissues except the supra- and interspinous ligaments are stripped from the spinous processes, laminae, and transverse processes. The posterior two-thirds of the facets are excised and grafted. B. A fusion from L4 to sacrum through midline approach is shown. Strips of graft from posterior ilium are laid from the sacrum to the transverse processes of L4. Care is taken to denude the outer face of the superior articular processes of L4 but not to damage the facet between L4 and L3. Reprinted from Ruge, D., Wiltse, L. L.: Chapter 15. In *Spinal Disorders: Diagnosis and Treatment.* Philadelphia, Lea & Febiger, 1977.

index finger can be inserted between these muscles down the apophyseal joint between L5 and S1.

The muscle fibers do not split cleanly at the L5 level but above this, a clear-cut cleavage plane can be found.

If a lumbosacral fusion is being done, care must be taken not to dissect too far cephalad or one will inadvertently expose the fourth lumbar vertebra. (There is a natural tendency to do this.) Two Gelpi retractors bent to a right angle at a point 2 inches from their tips are very good instruments for retracting the muscle. These are standard in most operating rooms or can be purchased from one of the large medical instrument companies.

The sacrospinalis is split only enough to expose the vertebrae to be fused. The top of the sacral ala should be denuded of soft tissue, but the posterior surface of the sacrum should not be denuded any more than is necessary for exposure because bone grafts will be placed in contact mainly with the top of the ala.

The laminae of the vertebra to be fused are exposed no more than 1.5 cm medial to the facet joints. The lumbar transverse processes should be denuded of soft tissue completely out to the tips and well around the superior and inferior borders. Especially in the child with high-grade slip, the iliolumbar and intertransverse ligaments are preserved carefully to prevent further slip. The spinal nerves are in front of the transverse processes and will not be injured provided the exposure is not continued anteriorly.

The lumbar arteries and veins, which pass just above the bases of the transverse processes and also at the angle of the medial point of the sacral ala, often bleed freely and can be difficult to stop with cautery. These bleeding "holes" should be plugged with a piece of Surgicel about 3 × 3 cm in size. Also, the vessels coming out of the superior sacral foramina may bleed rather profusely and these also can be staunched with Surgicel. This material should be removed later. However, no harm comes if a small wad of it is inadvertently left in. If the bleeding does not stop when ready to close, replace the Surgicel with Gelfoam and leave it in. Only bipolar cautery should be used in these areas as damage to the anterior rami can occur with unipolar cautery.[14]

Only the lateral surface of the superior articular processes of the topmost vertebra to be included in the fusion should be denuded. Care should be taken not to remove the capsule or to damage the adjacent joint, nor should one expose any part of the vertebra immediately above the fusion area. By observing these precautions, any tendency for the fusion to extend upward will be avoided.

Within the fusion area, the lateral surface of the superior articular process as well as the pars interarticularis and lamina to a point 1.5 cm medial to the facets are meticulously denuded of soft tissue. The spinous processes are not exposed, thereby preserving their ligamentous attachments and some of their blood supply. The facet joints within the fusion area are exposed carefully and the articular cartilage in the posterior two-thirds of each joint is removed. If a very loose element or spina bifida is present, this is not done.

A flap of bone from the back of the ala of the sacrum, based rostrally, is turned forward and cephalad to form a bridge to the transverse process of the fifth lumbar vertebra. Enough iliac graft can be obtained from one ilium through the same skin incision. The inner cortex is left intact. Cancellous bone is impacted between the denuded articular processes and strips of cancellous iliac and cortical bone are tamped very securely around the transverse processes, care being taken not to break them. The softer, pure cancellous bone is packed in first because it stays down well against the host bone. Cortical bone has a tendency to spring back from the transverse processes.

Postoperative Management

The patient is encouraged to get out of bed when he feels able to do so (usually in a day or two) and he is allowed to walk as much as he likes. It is preferred that he sit in a straight-backed chair and avoid deep overstuffed sofas for 2 months. A routine of exercises consisting of isometric abdominal and gluteal setting exercises is started 2 or

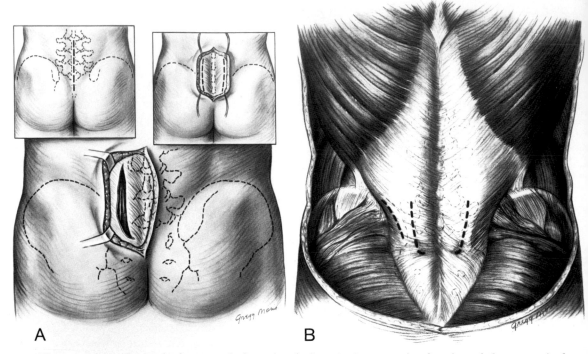

A   **B**

Figure 8.12. Paraspinal approach for spine fusion. A. A composite drawing of the paraspinal approach is shown. A midline skin incision is used but, once through the skin, the skin is pulled laterally and the fascia is cut two finger-breadths lateral to the midline. (Reprinted from Wiltse, L. L.: The paraspinal sacrospinalis-splitting approach to the lumbar spine. *Clin. Orthop. 91:*51–52, 1973.) B. The *dotted lines* show where the incision in the fascia are made. The line over the posterior superior iliac spine indicates the line of incision over the iliac crest if a bone graft is to be taken. One iliac crest will usually supply enough bone for both sides. C. Two Gelpi retractors seem to be the best instruments for retraction of the muscle. Note location of bone grafts after closure of the wound (*left*). D. The extent of bone graft used by the author is shown. Note that the graft covers the lateral surface of the superior articular process of the first sacral vertebra and that the joint between the fifth lumbar and the first sacral vertebra is fused. The joint between L4 and L5 is not injured but the graft extends onto the lateral aspect of the superior articular process of the fifth lumbar vertebra. An identical area is normally fused on the opposite side. Note: on the reader's right, a flap of bone is turned upward from the ala of the sacrum so it bridges the gap between the ala and the transverse process. (Reproduced from Wiltse, L. L.: Common problems of the lumbar spine: spondylolisthesis and its treatment. *J. Cont. Educ. Orthop.*, July, 1979.)

3 days after operation. All patients are trained to avoid motion of the low back by rolling like a log instead of twisting and by bending at the knees when stooping. Corsets and braces are not used for lumbosacral or L4 to sacrum fusions unless the patient prefers to wear one because no increase in the incidence of fusion has been observed with the use of these devices. Above L4, we prescribe a corset.

The Use of the Paraspinal Approach in Spondylolisthesis

The paraspinal approach described here has been especially valuable in children with spondylolisthesis. These children can be operated upon and allowed up immediately, in most cases. Because so few of the supporting ligaments have been cut vertically, no significant slip or sagittal rotation of the fifth lumbar vertebra has occurred in

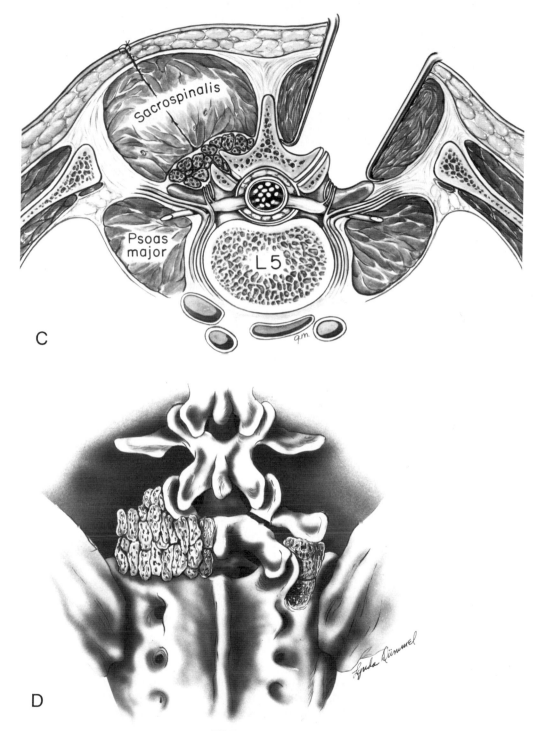

Figure 8.12. C and D.

our cases. The loose posterior element should not be removed in children unless we are planning to reduce the slip.

If the loose posterior element has been removed in a patient with spondylolisthesis, there is likelihood that some further slipping will occur. If the annulus has been incised for removal of a ruptured disc at the same level, in addition to removing the loose element, progression is virtually certain if the patient is allowed up before the fusion is solidified.[14]

When decompression of the cauda equina and nerve roots is indicated, it can be accomplished through this approach better than through the midline because this approach is centered almost directly over the region where the nerve root compression occurs. It is not necessary to do a complete laminectomy. With only a portion of the lamina removed, it is possible to trace the spinal nerve laterally and decompress it completely. If there are bony ossicles and a fibrocartilaginous mass associated with spondylolisthesis, they lie in the direct line of approach and easily can be removed.

In this connection, it is worth noting that, except in instances of high-grade slip, it is the fifth lumbar spinal nerve that is compressed in the presence of spondylolisthesis of the fifth lumbar vertebra. This may give the clinical picture of a ruptured disc at the interspace between the fourth and fifth lumbar vertebrae since an L4 disc usually compresses the L5 nerve root. In the rare case where the posterior border of the sacrum must be removed, a midline approach is better.

Spinal Fusion with the Gill Operation

We have not done a spinal fusion in conjunction with a Gill operation recently. This is because, if a proper Gill operation has been done, dura and nerves are exposed over a wide area and laying bone over these exposed nerves has not worked well. First, the fusion rate has not been good and second, the bone grows down around the nerves and seems to cause pain. If the leg pain is one-sided, then the L5 spinal nerve can be traced out laterally on the painful side as in Figure 8.13 and it is safe to fuse over this nerve with a limited decompression. On the other side, since no decompression has been done, a really good fusion can be done.

In spondylolisthesis in the adult, if the leg pain is not too severe, it is safer to do a fusion only, leaving the nerves untouched and risk having to do decompression later than it is to fuse over widely decompressed nerves.

The Unilateral Posterior Fusion

If back pain is present and most of the pain is in one leg, I would rather, through a paraspinal approach, totally decompress the one painful side and do a good fusion on the other side where there are intact bony structures (Fig. 8.14A and B).

Our unilateral fusions have done well where only one level needed to be fused and, in a small series, the fusion rate is very high. In fact, I know of no failures. If the surgeon is concerned about a fusion not becoming solid, he can add an interbody fusion and virtually assure success.

If the disc space is very narrow and osteoarthritic and the leg pain is mostly one-sided, the surgeon can do a unilateral Gill operation. To do a proper Gill operation it may be necessary to remove the caudal half of the pedicle and even the caudal half of the transverse process. One can fuse the other side through a paraspinal approach with a high degree of success.

Lumbar Interbody Fusion by the Anterior Route

Interbody fusions of the lumbar spine have been done for at least 50 years.[16, 17] This operation can be done either from in front through an abdominal incision or posteriorly by removing part of the lamina and retracting the cauda equina to one side as advocated by Cloward.[18-20] If an abdominal approach is decided upon, the surgeon has a further choice between a transperitoneal and a retroperitoneal approach. Several different techniques have been developed for both. I will describe here only the ones that I use at the present time.

If an interbody fusion is being considered, we usually do a discogram with a pain reproduction test. This is done as follows:

The patient is positioned on his side, and

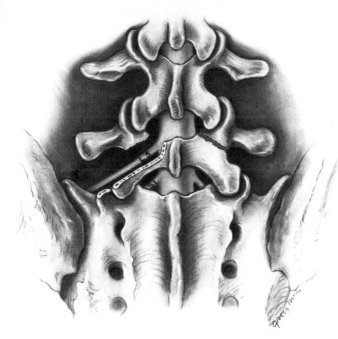

Figure 8.13. If the L5 spinal nerve is channelled as in this drawing, bone can be laid over the area from the sacral ala to the transverse process of L5, but it must be done with care or the bone will entrap the nerve.

local anesthesia is used, occasionally augmented by small amounts of intravenous Valium. The needles are inserted at a 45° angle, starting about 6–8 cm from the midline and entering the center of the disc. Two-plane x-ray is used to guide depth and angle determination. A small amount of Conray is injected to be sure the needle is properly placed. Then, more Conray is forced in under a fair amount of pressure. Often more volume is added by forcing in saline. The following situation may be found:

(1) A normal-appearing disc may be found on x-ray which is relatively painless on forced injection. This disc need not be included in the fusion.

(2) A degenerated disc may be seen on x-ray without reproduction of the patient's typical pain on injection. This disc space need not be included in the fusion.

(3) A degenerated disc may be seen on x-ray in which the patient's typical pain is reproduced on injection. Confirmatory information is gained if the pain is stopped dramatically by injection of 1.0 cc of 2% xylocaine. This disc space should be included in the fusion.

(4) Occasionally, several disc spaces are degenerated and all reproduce the typical pain. These patients are not candidates for spinal fusion if it is being done for pain alone.

Freebody Technique

Mr. Douglas Freebody of London has developed a technique which bears his name.[21] The details are as follows:

A midline incision and transperitoneal approach is made in the lower abdomen and the abdominal contents are moved out of the way. A catheter should be placed in the urinary bladder preoperatively to keep it as small as possible. A longitudinal incision is made in the posterior peritoneum overlying the vertebrae to be fused. Before this is done, the tissues overlying the bodies of L4, L5, and S1 are infiltrated with saline and epinephrine. This maneuver facilitates the identification of structures, permitting the presacral nerve and vessels to be moved laterally with a "pusher" as they pass over the sacral promontory.

Bleeding also is diminished by the epinephrine. Electrocoagulation should not be used here. If the bifurcation of the great

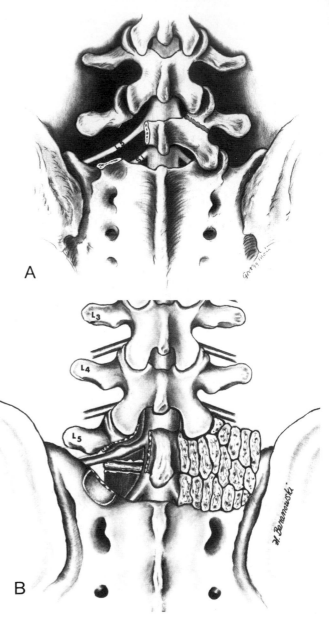

Figure 8.14. A. A type of total unilateral decompression is shown. (Reprinted from Wiltse, L. L.: The paraspinal sacrospinalis-splitting approach to the lumbar spine. *Clin. Orthop. 91:*48, 1973.) B. Unilateral fusion is shown.

vessels is high, the fifth disc can be approached between them. If bifurcation is low, the vessels can be retracted to the right after ligation of the left lumbar vessels which pass laterally around the vertebral bodies. The large vessels are carefully pushed over as far as possible to expose the disc and retractors are driven into place. A flap of annulus based to the right is then raised, and the disc is completely excised.

A portion of the end-plates is removed to raw bone.

Freebody removes a trap door from the front of the body of L5, and through this, access is gained to the top of S1. With a curette (or if the bone is too hard, a large drill), a hole is made through S1 to about the center of S2, perhaps 4 cm in depth. I have been making this hole using a $7/64$-inch guide pin under careful x-ray control. When the guide pin is properly placed, a large hip drill is passed over it, enlarging the hole further. A curette may be valuable here as well.

An osteoperiosteal flap then is lifted off the crest of the ilium and a full-thickness bone graft is removed from the top of the iliac crest at its thickest point. This graft is about 2.5 × 6 cm and is about the shape and size of a man's thumb. It is driven into the prepared slot across L5 into S1. The trap door is impacted back into the body of L5. The spaces on either side of the graft which had been occupied by disc tissue are curetted to bleeding bone and tamped full of cancellous bone. The patient is kept in a plaster bed for 6 weeks before ambulation is permitted and then only in a molded plastic jacket which he wears until the fusion appears solid.

Our results with the Freebody arthrodesis have been quite good. It has been used exclusively in cases of spondylolisthesis with high-grade slip. In some of our cases, nonunion has resulted even though the procedure seemed to have been performed well technically and the patients were immobilized postoperatively as recommended.

We prefer the transperitoneal approach when we must do an anterior fusion between L5 and S1 if there is high-grade slip. In such cases, it is virtually impossible to perform a satisfactory fusion of the L5, S1 interspace through a retroperitoneal approach.

Left Flank Approach

If we intend to go extraperitoneally, we have adopted a left flank incision, similar to that used for nephrectomy or sympathectomy when we intend to fuse the L3 or L4 but not the L5 level except in thin patients.

This approach is easily closed and is free of complications. The incision is an oblique one, halfway between the lower rib cage and the iliac crest. It is usually necessary to extend the incision an inch or two more medially than is required for sympathectomy. The incision then is carried through the external oblique, internal oblique, and transverse abdominal muscles. The vertical muscle bundles encountered generally have to be divided to obtain adequate exposure. To enter the retroperitoneal space, the posterior peritoneum is gently and bluntly dissected medially, a maneuver that exposes the anterior surface of the psoas muscle. The ureter has to be carefully mobilized so it is not damaged. Exposure is continued primarily by blunt dissection, mobilizing the vascular structures proximally and distally enough to expose the appropriate lumbar intervertebral space.

A troublesome problem is fragile lumbar veins which can bleed profusely if torn. Application of surgical hemoclips can be helpful in the control of small bleeders.[22] Another real advantage of this approach is that bone for the fusion can easily be removed without a separate skin incision.

Using Fibula Only

To fuse just one level, fibula alone is a good graft material. If two levels must be done, it is sometimes difficult to obtain enough bone from one leg. It is not advisable to remove fibula below the junction of its middle and lower thirds or less than 1½ inches from the top. When fibular struts are used, the vertical end-plates are excised and the bodies spread severely. The segments of fibula are sawed (Fig. 8.1) with a reciprocating saw and impacted into place securely. They are stood on end between the bodies. It is mandatory that these fibular grafts be held in place securely and that they be in a straight up-and-down position between the vertebral bodies. If they tip over, fusion will not occur.

Great care must be used in removing the fibula not to injure the superficial branch of the peroneal nerve. It lies on top of the fibular periosteum for 4–5 cm near the upper end. Use the Henry approach.[23] Do not separate the interosseous ligament below the junction of the lower and middle thirds.

Rib Grafts

Rib grafts are satisfactory in some situations. The rib grafts are cut to approximate length, the vertebral bodies are spread, and the segments are stood on end between the bodies. Rib graft is much weaker than fibula but has good osteogenic potential.

Also, rib grafts are used to good advantage in cases of tuberculosis when cavities in the vertebral bodies must be filled with bone. Often rib portions are resected in the approach in these cases, furnishing a ready source of grafting materials.

Iliac Grafts

Iliac grafts placed as shown in Figure 8.2 are used occasionally. I prefer these where it is not necessary to have severe separation of the bodies, iliac bone being somewhat soft. Our success rate of fusion has not been as good as with fibula but Goldner[24] believes that, if a very large volume of iliac graft material can be placed, as in Figure 8.2, the success rate will be high. He occasionally utilizes as many as five of these horseshoe shaped grafts.

Dowel Grafts

Harmon[16] has described the use of a single large dowel for interbody fusion. Recently, Crock[25] has described a technique of using a double-dowel graft. These grafts are taken from the ilium with special instruments. This operation is technically a very elegant procedure when done as described by Dr. Crock.

Dr. Crock now uses the Frazer exposure which is described as follows:

The incision runs obliquely from the midline parallel with the iliac crest, approximately midway between the umbilicus and symphysis pubis, upwards and laterally for about 8–9 cm. Then, the exposure through this skin incision is in the line of the fibers of the external oblique. The external oblique fibers then are split from the level of the lateral edge of the rectus sheath laterally over the desired length of the incision. The edges of the external oblique are then retracted and these expose the fibers of the internal oblique which are running upwards and medially from the iliac crest. The fibers of the internal oblique now are split just lateral to the lateral edge of the rectus sheath and these fibers are retracted to expose beneath them the fibers of the transverse abdominus running obliquely in relation to the internal oblique fibers.

Now by splitting the internal oblique at the same level, the extraperitoneal space is entered. Once this has been done, a pair of scissors is used to make a vertical incision just inside the lateral edge of the rectus sheath running downward for a distance of 5–6 cm. This creates a flap of transversalis and internal oblique which can be turned downward and laterally, allowing for easy and wide extraperitoneal exposure of the lumbar spine.

I especially like the interbody fusion in situations where only one space is involved. It is ideal for cases of discogenic vertebral sclerosis.[25] Also, it can be used in cases where there has been failure of fusion posteriorly and the acceptance test indicates that that is the level causing the pain.

No one should attempt an anterior interbody fusion of the lumbar spine without special retractors. Several types have been designed.

Finally, I would warn that the surgeon who only occasionally does an anterior lumbar fusion is likely to find that his nonunion rate is unacceptably high.

Lumbar Interbody Fusion by the Posterior Route

Cloward has described a method of interbody fusion through a posterior midline approach.[18–20] In this operation, the laminae are approached as for a classic laminectomy. The interspinous ligament and the margins of the adjacent spinous processes are removed to permit the insertion of a special vertebral spreader. About one-half of the adjacent laminal edge is removed along with the medial portion of the facets.

The cauda equina is retracted halfway to one side. The cortical surfaces of the adjacent vertebral bodies are removed in a straight, even fashion as far as raw bleeding bone.[18-20]

Full-thickness iliac grafts, autogenous or homogenous, then are driven into the place, two on each side, making a total of four to fill the disc space completely. The wound is closed routinely and the patient is permitted out of bed when able.

The Cloward technique or modifications[26] are being used with increasing frequency. The major disadvantage of the Cloward technique is that, being a posterior approach, one has to pull the dura over to the side a moderate amount. Dr. Cloward believes that this is not a disadvantage and that his results have been good. Certainly from a theoretical standpoint, the Cloward technique has advantages. At the moment, I am re-evaluating the Cloward method[18-20] and use it occasionally. Great care should be used in retracting the dura and its contents. I have never used the Cloward procedure above the L4 space but others have no hesitancy in putting grafts at L3. Some cases of partial paralysis have been reported from grafting at too high a level, especially in the case of a low conus. The technique is, of course, good when posterior decompression and fusion are both necessary, but Murphy[27] claims that the fusion rate is low when all posterior support has been removed.

Postoperative Care Following Lumbar Interbody Fusion

Except in the case of the Freebody operation, we permit ambulation just a few days after operation. We do not normally use a brace but, if concerned about the stability of the graft, a brace may be prescribed.

Testing the Stability of the Fusion

The question of whether the fusion is or is not solid is always troublesome. In cases of anterior interbody fusion, we must see trabeculae crossing the interspace to be sure of fusion, but we do not have this guide in posterior fusions. In either case, we use lateral views of flexion and extension bending films with the patient lying down. Intravenous demerol is given if pain is a limiting factor.

Lines are drawn with wax pencil over the bony landmarks and these lines are superimposed over a bright light. In taking the films, a square is laid against the bony prominences to be sure that the patient is not twisting while exposures are made during flexion and extension. We believe that films taken with the patient lying down are of better quality and superimpose better than if taken standing.

Unfortunately, in the patient who has had multiple back operations and still has pain and pseudarthrosis, even getting a solid fusion often does not relieve the pain. What then is the place of lumbar fusion in the treatment of low back pain? We use it in the patient who fulfills the following criteria:

(1) There is evidence that the levels above the area of contemplated fusion are reasonably normal.

(2) There are favorable psychologic studies.

(3) The patient is in good general health and under 65 years of age (or 70 in psychologically young people). I limit the age because older people are probably best advised to limit their activities and not be fused.

(4) There is positive pain reproduction in the test at the level or levels to be fused, especially in cases of pseudarthrosis.

(5) Of course, we use it where real instability is likely to be a problem.

Spinal Stenosis Following Lumbar Spinal Fusion

I have not seen spinal stenosis develop secondary to anterior interbody fusion, nor have I seen spinal stenosis develop after posterior fusion except (1) at the top of the fusion mass, (2) at a point of pseudoarthrosis, or (3) where bone graft has been laid over areas of decompression. If a laminectomy has been done and then bone graft laid over the open laminectomy site, ingrowth does occur. There are several months before the fusion becomes solid and, during this time, when there is motion, bone may grow in. I have not seen spinal stenosis develop in the sacral canal postfusion. Therefore, I conclude that feathering the back of the sacrum or an intact lamina does not cause bone to grow anteriorly. However, if pseudoarthrosis exists for several years underneath a fusion, bone can certainly grow anteriorly and block the canal. The fusion may finally become solid and we are erroneously led to believe the bone grew forward from an intact lamina.

Several times, where we have done a one-level fusion in the adult for spondylolisthesis, we have traced the L5 nerve far out laterally, then laid bone from the sacral ala to the transverse process of L5, thus necessarily bridging an exposed nerve. Bone will grow around the nerve in this situation. For this reason, we have not done this in recent years.

If, in the case of spondylolisthesis, pain down the legs is not very severe, do a spinal fusion without any decompression. If the pain in the legs continues, then do a decompression as a secondary procedure after the fusion is solid. Either one or both sides can be easily decompressed if a wide transverse process fusion has been obtained. If the leg pain is very severe, the surgeon can do a fusion with the express understanding that a decompression of the nerve will be done after the fusion is solid which of course will be 8–10 months.

Isolated Disc Resorption and Discogenic Vertebral Sclerosis[28, 29]

Crock has described isolated disc resorption. There is also a closely related type of isolated disc disease which has been called discogenic vertebral sclerosis.[2] We have seen this condition two or three times a

year for the past many years. In these cases, the disc (L4, but also other levels) just seems to disappear. Sclerosis of the contiguous surfaces of the body develops. This sclerosis may travel into the vertebral body by 2–3 cm.

Pain in the back without leg pain is characteristic. We have generally done a needle biopsy and culture before operation since a real possibility of infection is present. On two occasions, we have cultured out staphylococcus epidermidis. We have followed with interbody fusion, using fibula and recently, ilium. The pain relief has been dramatic in most cases and so far, there have been no failures of fusion in the fibular grafts. Our iliac grafts are too recent to be sure of the rate of fusion.

We have not done this procedure where there has been significant leg pain. It is likely that pain relief would be very good even in the presence of leg pain because the disc is removed and the bodies jacked apart. The Cloward operation ought to be ideal in this last situation.

SUMMARY

In deciding whether or not to fuse, we must remember the admonition that spinal fusion should be done for instability and decompression for spinal nerve pressure. As our knowledge increases and our diagnostic skills improve, we should be able to learn to fuse the appropriate case primarily, and thus, save the patient an extra operation. The 1970's was the decade of decompression. Now lumbar spine surgeons seem to be swinging back to doing more fusions. A veritable smorgasbord of choices of techniques has been developed. Yet none are ideal and the failure rate of solid arthrodesis is still distressingly high. Radical unstabilizing decompression alone is certainly not the answer. Perhaps the decade of the 1980's will be the one during which we learn how and when to fuse.

As the population gets older, we see more and more people in their mid-60's very severely disabled and occasionally even wheelchair-bound because of lumbar spine disease. Often, these patients have lumbar scoliosis which we note (on reviewing old x-rays) was mild 10 years ago but has been increasing at the rate of a degree or two per year. Severe degenerative disc disease, often with marked rotation of one vertebra on the other in the midlumbar area, is the rule. If a myelogram is done, extreme spinal stenosis is noted. If a massive decompression is done, the leg pain may be relieved but the back pain most often is increased and even the leg pain will return in 8–12 months. Added to this, after the massive unstabilizing operation posteriorly, scoliosis and rotation increase much more rapidly because of loss of the posterior elements.

We must learn a practical method for fusing several levels in these people. Harrington rods and their various modifications such as the Lugue system along with the modifications of the Dwyer fusion offer possibilities. Perhaps new methods of stimulating bone formation can be used in conjunction with fusion. We still have the problem of where to get enough bone for this kind of massive arthrodesis. The bone substitutes are on the horizon and may be practical in the next few years.

Finally, I do not believe that a spinal fusion is often necessary in association with a simple laminectomy done for a ruptured disc unless there is some other cause for instability.

References

1. Williams, J. L., Moller, G. A., O'Rourke, T. L.: Pseudoinfection of the intervertebral disc and adjacent vertebrae. *Am. J. Roentgen. 103:*611, 1968.
2. Crock, H. V.: Isolated lumbar disc resorption as a cause of nerve root canal stenosis. *Clin. Orthop. 115:*109, 1976.
3. Barr, J. S.: Lumbar disc lesions in retrospect and prospect. Address tape recorded at the meeting of the Officers' Club, San Diego Naval Hospital, May 15, 1961. *Clin. Orthop. 129:*4, 1977.
4. Mixter, W. J., Barr, J. S.: Rupture of the intervertebral disc with involvement of the spinal canal. *N. Engl. J. Med. 211:*210, 1934.
5. McElroy, K. D.: Lumbosacral fusion by bilateral-lateral technique. Proceedings of the American Academy of Orthopaedic Surgeons. *J. Bone Joint Surg. 43-A:*918, 1961.
6. Caldwell, G. A., Sheppard, W. B.: Criteria for spine fusion following removal of a protruded nucleus pulposus. *J. Bone Joint Surg. 30A:*971–977, 1948.
7. Reynolds, J. B., Wiltse, L. L.: Surgical treatment of degenerative spondylolisthesis. *Spine 4:*148, 1979.
8. DePalma, A., Rothman, R.: The nature of pseudarthrosis. *Clin. Orthop. 59:*113, 1968.
9. Sacks, S.: Symposium on the spine. *Orthop. Clin. N. A. 6(1):*275, 1975.
10. Flynn, J. C.: Anterior lumbar interbody fusion. Paper presented at American Academy Orthopedic Surg. Institute course, Orlando, Florida, Dec. 5, 1980.
11. Rosomoff, H. H.: Bony encroachment of the lumbar spine: a cause of low back surgery failure. *J. Fla. Med. Assoc. 63:*884, 1976.
12. Mensor, M. D., Duvall, G.: Absence of motion at the 4th and 5th lumbar interspaces in patients with and without low back pain. *J. Bone Joint Surg. 41-A:*1047, 1959.
13. Wiltse, L. L., Bateman, J. G., Hutchinson, R. J.: The paraspinal sacrospinalis-splitting approach to the lumbar spine. *J. Bone Joint Surg. 91:*51, 1968.
14. Macnab, I., Dall, C.: The blood supply of the lumbar spine and its application to the technic of intertransverse lumbar fusions. *J. Bone Joint Surg. 53-B:*628, 1971.
15. Wiltse, L. L., Hutchinson, R. H.: The surgical treatment of spondylolisthesis. *Clin. Orthop. 35:*116, 1964.
16. Harmon, P. D.: Anterior extraperitoneal lumbar disc excision and vertebral body fusion. *Clin. Orthop. 18:*169, 1960.
17. Harmon, P. D.: Anterior disc excision and fusion of the lumbar vertebral bodies: a review of diagnostic testing with operative results in more than 700 cases. *J. Intern. Coll. Surg. 40:*572, 1963.
18. Cloward, R. B.: The treatment of ruptured intervertebral discs by vertebral body fusion. *Ann. Surg. 136:*987–992, 1952.
19. Cloward, R. B.: The treatment of ruptured lumbar intervertebral discs by vertebral body fusion. Indications, techniques, after care. *J. Neurosurg. 10:*154, 1953.
20. Cloward, R. B.: Lesion of the intervertebral discs and their treatment by interbody fusion methods. *Clin. Orthop. 27:*51–77, 1963.
21. Freebody, D., Bedall, R., Taulor, R. D.: Anterior transperitoneal lumbar fusion. *J. Bone Joint Surg. 53B:*617, 1971.
22. Hickman, E.: Personal Communication, 1973.
23. Henry, M. O.: Homografts in orthopedic surgery. *J. Bone Joint Surg. 30-A:*70, 1948.
24. Goldner, L.: Personal Communication, Feb. 1, 1979.
25. Crock, H. V.: Recommended incision as described

by Robert Frazer from Flinders University, South Australia, for the exposure by extraperitoneal approach to the lower lumbar spine. Personal Communication, February 1981.

26. Lin, Paul M.: Posterior lumbar interbody fusion. Paper presented at the Lumbar Spine Surgery Seminar, Gainesville, FL, April, 1980.

27. Murphy, Robert: Personal Communication, February 1981.

28. Demos, C. D.: Benign vertebral sclerosis. *Orthopaedics, 4(1):*72, 1981.

29. Sauser, D. D., Goldman, A. B., Kaye, J. J.: Discogenic vertebral sclerosis. *J. Can. Assoc. Radiolog.* *29:*44, March 1978.

9

Chemonucleolysis

It is indeed a rare occurrence in medicine that a form of treatment, radically different from the current and established mode of therapy, is introduced in the management of a specific disease entity. As its use gains wider acceptance and early good results are confirmed and sustained, it becomes, in due course, a standard procedure. Such has been the history of chemonucleolysis.

Although Mixter and Barr[1] identified herniations of the nucleus pulposus as a disease entity in 1934, it was not until 1948 that Lindbloom[2] reported the first diagnostic discogram. In 1959, the concept of chemical dissolution of the nucleus pulposus was introduced by Carl Hirsch.[3] Two years later, Lyman Smith started experimental studies in rabbits by injecting chymopapain into the disc.[4] His first clinical results were published in 1964.[5] The initial response of practicing orthopaedic surgeons and neurosurgeons was modest; by 1975, well over 16,000 patients had been treated by this method in the United States of America. The Canadian Health Protection Board approved the use of chymopapain in 1971. Presently, approximately 4000 cases are done annually in Canada. It also is accepted widely in other countries, including Great Britain, France, Belgium, Italy, Japan, and the USSR.

CHYMOPAPAIN

Chymopapain is one of three proteolytic enzymes that can be extracted from the latex of the tropical fruit, Carica papaya. Chymopapain is a sulfur-containing enzyme; therefore, to promote activity and stability, reducing agents such as cysteine

are required to maintain the sulfur in sulfhydryl form. High activity is achieved only in the presence of chelating agents such as sodium EDTA. It is extremely thermolabile and, as such, it should be kept refrigerated and only reconstituted immediately before its use for it will lose 25% of its potency during each hour exposed to room temperature.[6]

TOXICOLOGY

Chymopapain is the safest and most specific of all the enzymes capable of dissolving the nucleus pulposus. Fortunately, there is a marked difference between the discolytic and toxic dose. In the vertebrates, the higher one proceeds up the phylogenetic scale, the less toxic the enzyme becomes when injected intravenously on a weight basis. The toxicity is much higher in the mouse, less in the rabbit, and minimal in man.[7] It is understandable that, in man, the toxicity increases as one proceeds in the cophalad direction. For this reason, chemonucleolysis is contraindicated in the management of cervical disc disease. However, as it is well known, herniations of the nucleus pulposus are considerably less of a problem in the cervical spine.

According to studies carried out in experimental animals,[8] chymopapain has no affect on ligament, muscle, nerve, and epidural tissue. The adverse effects on meninges, epidural and neural tissue described by Shealy and Rydevik et al.[9, 10] have not been confirmed by others, including MacNab et al.[11] and Ford.[12] Large doses administered intrathecally in the experimental animal are highly toxic. Fatal subarachnoid hemorrhages result, due to the rupture of pial and arachnoid vessels.[13, 14]

MECHANISM OF ACTION

When injected intradiscally, the sole action of chymopapain is limited to the nucleus pulposus. It has virtually no effect on the annulus fibrosus. Both in vitro and in vivo studies[15, 16] showed that chymopapain exerts a hydrolytic effect on the noncollagenous protein bonds that interconnect long chain mucopolysaccharides; this chondromucoprotein is responsible for the water-retaining capability of the nucleus pulposus. Lyman Smith postulated that the intradiscal pressure is lowered by rapidly decreasing the water content of the disc, abolishing posterior tenting of the neural structures.[17, 18] It has been our experience that in a very high proportion of patients, the disabling sciatica virtually disappears by the time the action of the anesthetic has worn off. When an obvious muscular weakness of the extensor hallucis longus or the triceps surae is present, the muscle strength rapidly returns. Although the mechanism is obscure, it seems that after chymopapain injection, intradiscal pressure decreases rapidly and tension on the nerve root is immediately relieved. Certainly, this is evidenced clinically, however the myelographic picture remains unchanged for a long period of time. It is difficult to believe that the intradiscal pressure has decreased rapidly enough to relieve immediately the tension on the nerve root. Intradiscal pressure measurements before chemonucleolysis and 1 hour after disc dissolution are needed for further clarification.

The alkaline wash theory[12] has been suggested as a possible explanation for the immediate relief of pain following chemonucleolysis. By the introduction of an alkaline substance such as chymopapain, cysteine, and sodium EDTA into the nucleus pulposus, the free hydrogen ions present in the abnormal disc are neutralized. Therefore, stimulation of afferent pain-transmitting fibers does not occur. The increase in intradiscal pH also may explain why one can observe temporary symptomatic improvement following the injection of steroids into the nucleus pulposus.

SELECTION OF PATIENTS FOR CHEMONUCLEOLYSIS

Chemonucleolysis is indicated in the treatment of back pain and sciatica secondary to lumbar disc herniation which has failed to respond to an adequate trial of conservative therapy. Its use should be restricted to patients who have come to a point where they would consider surgery as the next step in their management.

It soon becomes apparent to the practicing surgeon that there are two readily distinguishable groups of patients with back pain and sciatica. The first and largest group includes patients who are typically middle-aged, more commonly female, and in relatively poor physical condition. A long-standing history of intermittent low back pain and discogenic sciatica can be elicited. Physical findings, particularly those of root compression, are conspicuously absent. It is suggested that these patients should be managed conservatively as they are poor candidates for surgery or chemonucleolysis.

The second group of patients comprises those with an acute lumbar disc herniation. Typically, the patient is between the ages of 20 and 50 years, more commonly male, and gives a history of back pain and sciatica either with or without antecedent lumbar trauma. The sciatic pain is usually more disabling than the associated back pain. Physical findings demonstrate all the signs of a herniated nucleus pulposus with root compression. If these patients fail to respond to conservative treatment, they should be considered good candidates for chemonucleolysis.

A recent review of the author's first 373 patients, followed for a minimum of 1 year, showed that patients who obtained the best results with chemonucleolysis were those who gave the typical history of acute lumbar disc herniation as described previously.[19] Physical findings of particular importance are as follows: restricted forward flexion of the lumbar spine with flexion of the symptomatic leg at the knee on this maneuver; a drift of the spine away from or towards the side of sciatica; weakened toe or heel walk on the symptomatic side, and a strongly positive Lasegue test. In this series, only 35% of patients demonstrated a definite neurologic deficit. Plain x-rays of the lumbar spine were either normal or revealed only minor changes of degenerative disc disease at one or two levels. Almost one-half of the disc herniations demonstrated discographically were at levels which appeared completely normal on plain films.

Three absolute criteria were met by all patients who underwent chemonucleolysis:

(1) *Pain.* Back and/or leg pain, characteristic of degenerative disc disease, was present.

(2) *Course of conservative therapy.* Each patient had a minimum of 2 weeks of bed rest, administration of muscle relaxants and anti-inflammatory agents, followed by a course of physiotherapy. Of the cases treated, 90% had persistent symptoms for longer than 12 weeks, despite these maneuvers.

(3) *Discographic evidence of a lumbar disc herniation.* This is described later in this chapter.

In addition to the preceding, all of the patients have met at least two of the following three criteria:

(1) *limitation of back flexion* (less than 45°) with or without muscle spasm;

(2) *limitation of straight leg raising* (less than 90°) with pain;

(3) *neurologic deficit:* (a) diminished or absent sensation in the L4, L5, or S1 dermatome, (b) diminished or absent reflexes.

Specific groups of patients warrant particular mention as to their suitability for chemonucleolysis.

1. *Previous low back surgery* is not a contraindication for chemonucleolysis as such; however, one has to be extremely selective. A patient must have had symptomatic improvement after lumbar disc surgery and then experienced a recurrence at the level previously operated upon, at the level above a solid fusion, or at a new level. The prognosis in these cases is guarded, although satisfactory results have been reported by several authors in up to 50% of these patients.[20, 21] In this series, the author has achieved a 60% success rate in this type of patient.

2. *Disc protrusions in adolescence* are an uncommon clinical situation. To date, nine such patients have been treated. In this type of patient, the results from surgical procedures may be unsatisfactory,[22, 23] whereas after chemonucleolysis, they are very gratifying.

3. *In patients with major neurologic deficits,* chemonucleolysis is contraindicated. Patients with a cauda equina syndrome require rapid surgical decompression. However, it may be stated that chemonucleolysis is the treatment of choice in the management of a drop foot secondary to a herniated lumbar disc. In all patients with drop feet (eight cases of unilateral and one case of bilateral drop feet), the author has noted relief of paralysis after chemical dissolution of the disc.

4. *Extruded disc* is a diagnosis that can be confirmed only at the time of surgery. However, occasionally, we may see a patient where the diagnosis can presumably be made on clinical and radiologic grounds. The patients complain of neurogenic sciatica and have a strongly positive Lasegue sign that can be elicited on the symptomatic side, including crossed-leg reference. In these cases, the myelogram shows an obstruction of the contrast column with a disc fragment positioned posteriorly to the vertebral body. These patients have been classified by several investigators as ideal candidates for chemonucleolysis[24, 25] a finding confirmed in this series.

The question of the mechanism of dissolution of extruded discs frequently arises. As the nucleus pulposus herniates through a radial tear in the annulus and ultimately extrudes through the outer lamella of the annulus to lie in the extradural space, it is possible that the enzyme will follow the route of least resistance. Failure of chemonucleolysis should be expected only if the disc has been extruded for a prolonged period of time and where it has been walled off with fibrous tissue. This condition results in a sequestered disc fragment for which surgical excision is necessary. It is impossible to predict preoperatively which extruded disc fragment is already sequestered. Chemonucleolysis should be tried in the hope that surgery may be avoided.

5. *Chemonucleolysis should not be used* in women who are pregnant nor in individuals who have a known allergy to papaya or its derivatives. Although the number of sensitized patients is very small, it is unfortunate that a skin test is not available at the present time to assess patient sensitivity to the enzyme.

6. *Repeat chemonucleolysis.* In the present series, there are seven patients who have undergone repeat chemonucleolysis procedures with a satisfactory result. I have noted in the course of follow-up studies that re-expansion of the disc space height to its prechemonucleolysis state is occasionally observed in young individuals (Fig. 9.1A, B, and C). I have suggested re-injecting the disc if, after the first procedure, the patient had an excellent result and the recurrence has taken place some years later. In the seven patients of my series, the earliest time interval between the original procedure and the reinjection was 2.5 years and the longest was 16 years.

TECHNIQUE OF CHEMONUCLEOLYSIS

The author has been actively using chymopapain since 1973. Chemonucleolysis is considered to be an in-patient procedure and the routine workup of the patient is identical to that used before laminectomy. The following steps in technique should be emphasized:

(1) *General anesthesia* is routinely administered at our institution. The most serious, though infrequent, complication after chemonucleolysis is an anaphylactic reaction occurring within the 15 minutes after the injection of the enzyme. The usual manifestations are pulmonary and cardiovascular in nature. With endotracheal intubation, an adequate airway can be maintained to counteract the bronchial spasm, should it ensue. An intravenous line is maintained to replace fluids and to administer medications in the event of cardiovascular collapse. General anesthesia will attenuate serious complications and will not mask the symptoms of an anaphylactic reaction. It should be emphasized that halothane anesthesia should not be used. Halothane will sensitize the myocardium to catecholamines,[26, 27] the drug of choice in the event of an anaphylactic reaction.[28]

(2) *Positioning of the patient* is most important. Meticulous attention to details of positioning is essential if one is to reach the center of the nucleus pulposus with ease and regularity. The patient may be placed in the left or the right lateral decubitus position, depending on the physical setup of the operating or x-ray room. We routinely use the left lateral decubitus position, centering the spine using biplane image intensification. The anteroposterior view is monitored on a Phillips BV 22 image intensifier and the lateral view is obtained on a Phillips angiogram table with a floating table top. A cushion is placed under the patient's left flank and inflated to the point where the spine is straight (Fig. 9.2). A convexity or a concavity of the spine should be avoided when positioning the patient. This may hinder the entry of the needle into the disc at any level and it could render entry impossible at the L5-S1 disc space. The patient is held in position with adhesive tape. Particular attention is paid to

assure that the spinous process bisects the pedicles, preferably at all five lumbar vertebrae, when viewed on cross-table anteroposterior fluoroscopy (Fig. 9.3).

DISCOGRAPHY

Discography is of primary importance for chemonucleolysis. If the needles are not properly positioned in the nucleus pulposus, delivery of the enzyme to the correct location is impossible and the procedure will result in failure. It is generally agreed that 90% of disc herniations occur at the functioning lower two levels of the lumbar spine. For this reason, it has been our prac-

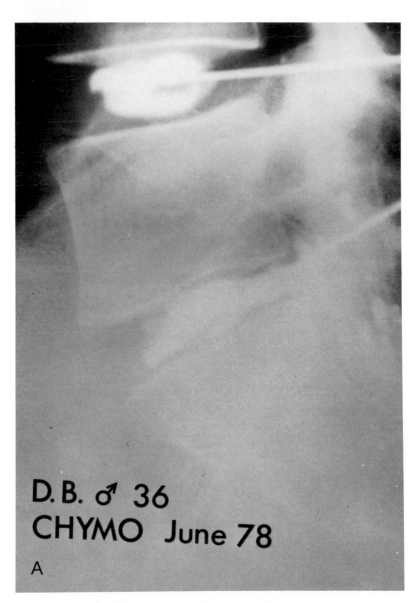

Figure 9.1. A. Disc re-expansion of L5-S1 chemonucleolysis in June 1978 is shown. B. At four months postchemonucleolysis, note the narrowing of the L5-S1 disc space. C. Chemonucleolysis is repeated 29 months after the first procedure; note re-expansion of L5-S1 disc.

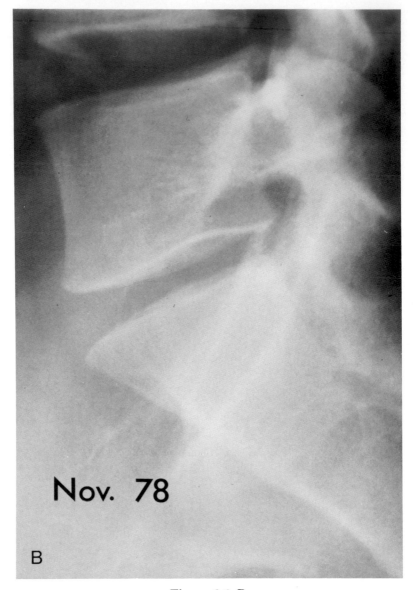

Figure 9.1. B.

tice to routinely carry out discographic examinations of the L4–5 and L5-S1 disc spaces. The L3–4 space only is examined if the clinical picture suggests involvement at this level or if there is myelographic evidence of a disc herniation at this space.

We believe that it is advisable to explain the evolution of the above protocol. When first using the procedure, the lumbar spine was approached in the same way as one would approach the lumbar spine surgically in the management of herniated lumbar discs. In other words, a myelogram first was performed, followed by a discographic examination at the level of the myelographic defect. If the herniation was demonstrated discographically, this level would be treated by chemonucleolysis. Two levels would be examined discographically only if the myelogram demonstrated a protrusion at both levels. This approach was adopted in the initial cases because of general belief that

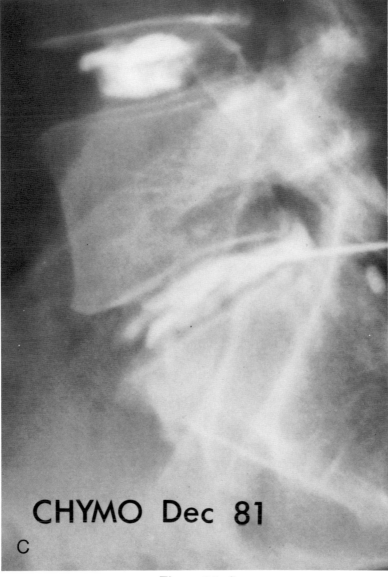

CHYMO Dec 81

C

Figure 9.1. C.

results were poor in patients who had two- and three-level discectomies compared to those in which only one level was involved.

In subsequent review of early cases, it became apparent that in patients who underwent two-level chemonucleolysis, the results were almost as good as in those with single level injections. Patients with isolated L4–5 lesions did not do as well as those with isolated L5-S1 disc herniations. Even though the number of cases was small, patients in which three-level chemonucleolysis was performed constituted the group in which the results almost equalled the results of single level injections. It is very tempting to assume that if a two-level herniation is seen on the myelogram that the largest herniation is causing all the symptoms, but this does not seem to be the case. We cannot be certain that the smaller disc protrusion is not a major contributing factor to the patient's symptoms.

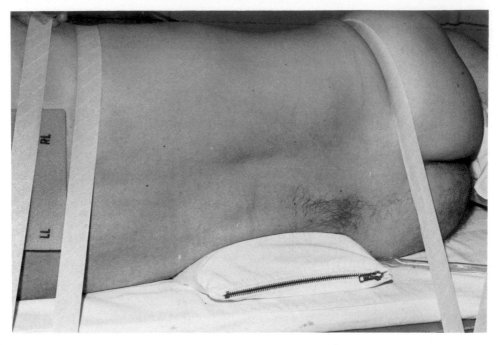

Figure 9.2. Positioning: the patient is in the left lateral decubitus position and held with tape. Inflatable cushion is placed under left flank.

By examining Figure 9.4, it appears that the number of L4–5, L5-S1, and multiple level protrusions is relatively constant for each decade of life. If this observation is true, it does not confirm the general impression that degeneration begins at the L5-S1 disc space and proceeds in the cephalad direction with advancing age.

Many authors stress the importance of the Saline Acceptance Test.[33] I have found this test to be of little value because the results are often equivocal when the patient is sedated. The procedure is more uncomfortable than a myelogram and may induce the patient to move, thereby making lateral discography much more difficult.

For the reasons previously outlined, the patient should be anesthetized, enhancing the ease of performing a very straight forward procedure. The injection of chymopapain at all involved levels seems mandatory in order to obtain the optimal result.

Insertion of the needle must be precise. The patient's right flank is prepared and draped as a sterile field. A point 8 cm lateral to the spinous process is marked. A 6-inch spinal needle (18 gauge with stylet) is introduced at an angle approximating 60° (Fig. 9.5). This angle actually varies, depending on the size of the patient.

The needle is advanced slowly in a stop-go fashion, constantly verifying the position of the tip in the anteroposterior and the lateral planes. The L4–5 disc is entered first and its position is confirmed in two planes. Subsequently, the L5-S1 disc is approached from the same point, directing the needle 30° caudad (Fig. 9.6A and B).

Bony vertebral elements are the major obstacles to the proper placement of the needles. Difficulties in this respect may be minimized by selecting the correct skin entry point. This is done by placing the needle over the flank under image intensification and then attempting to position the needle parallel to the end-plates of the disc space, as viewed on the lateral plane. Once this has been achieved, an imaginary line is

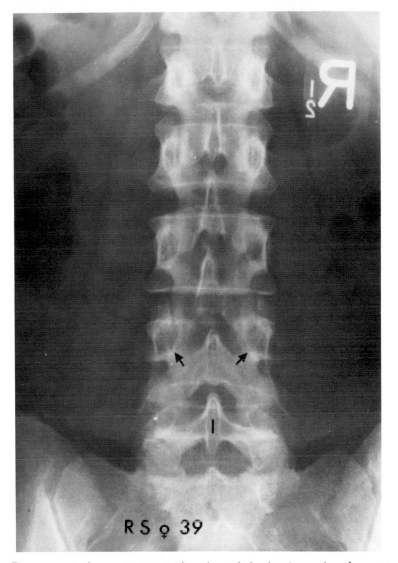

Figure 9.3. Proper centering: anteroposterior view of the lumbar spine demonstrates proper centering. Notice that the spinous process of L4 is equidistant from both pedicles.

dropped from the end of the needle to the point 8 cm lateral to the spinous process. This extremely simple preliminary step greatly facilitates the technique for lateral discography (Fig. 9.7).

Technical difficulties are encountered most often at the L5-S1 disc. Four situations warrant particular attention:

(1) *Degeneration of the disc space with marked narrowing* may make penetration extremely difficult. In such an instance, we would use a 3-inch, 18-gauge spinal needle with stylet as a guide in approaching the disc. Once the needle is near the annulus, a 6-inch, 22-gauge spinal needle with stylet is inserted through the 3-inch guide needle to enter the nucleus pulposus.

(2) *A very deep-seated L5 vertebra* frequently makes a lateral approach to the L5-S1 disc impossible. Once the radiologic picture is assessed and a difficulty is encountered in the lateral approach, we should

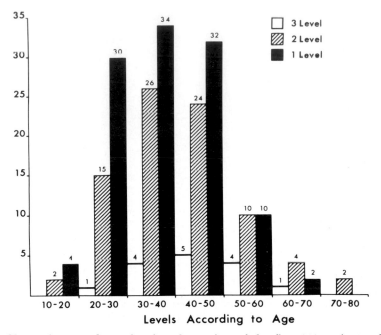

Figure 9.4. Shown is an early study after the review of the first 210 patients who underwent chemonucleolysis. This demonstrates that although there is a slightly higher ratio of multiple level disc degenerations and herniations in the older age group, this really only becomes apparent after the fifth decade. This graph also underlines the fact that discography should be carried out routinely at the L4–5 and L5-S1 disc spaces.

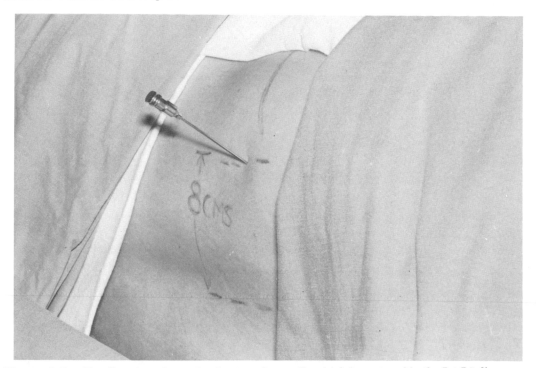

Figure 9.5. Needle entry: the angle of entry of a needle which is centered in the L4-L5 disc space is shown.

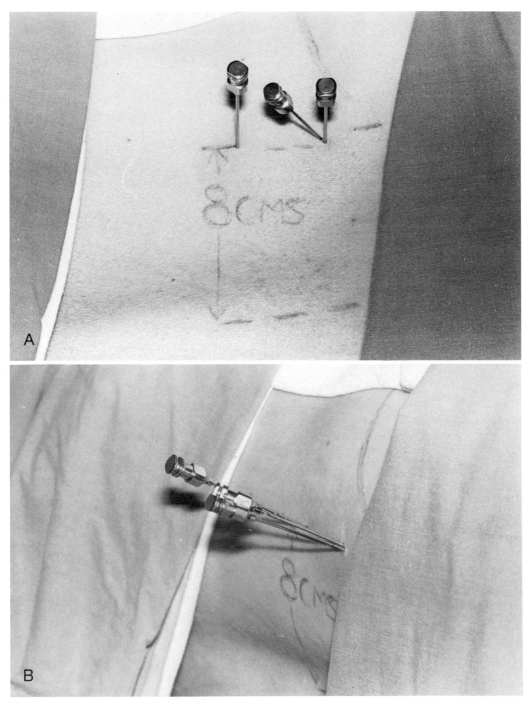

Figure 9.6.   A. The position of needles for three-level lateral discography is shown. The needle on the *left* is centered in the L3–4 disc space. The needle on the far *right* is centered in the L4–5 disc space. Notice the 30° angle of the needle which is centered in the L5-S1 disc space. B. Centered needles: this lateral view depicts needles centered in the L3–4, L4–5, and L5-S1 disc spaces.

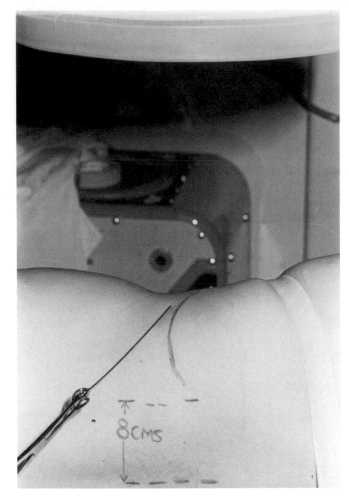

Figure 9.7.   Skin entry point to facilitate disc entry: the draping of this patient has been omitted to more easily demonstrate the preliminary step used to determine the precise skin entry point to facilitate disc entry.

proceed immediately with a posterior transdural approach to the L5-S1 disc space. The author has resorted to the posterior approach in approximately 5% of L5-S1 discograms.

(3) *Lumbarization of the S1 vertebra or sacralization of the L5 vertebra* may be encountered. If there is articulation of at least one transverse process with the sacrum, an assumption can be made that this disc level is not contributing to the patient's symptoms. The motion segment of L5-S1 is inherently stable precluding herniation of the nucleus pulposus.

(4) *Asymmetry of the transverse processes* can present difficulties. Minor developmental anomalies frequently can be ob-

served at the lumbosacral junction and, occasionally, a marked difference in the length and width of the transverse processes of the L5 vertebra may be present. If we encounter an abnormally long or a wide transverse process on the right side of the L5 vertebra, lateral discography from the left side should be considered in order to facilitate entry into the nucleus of L5-S1.

Once the needle has been centered in the disc, a discographic examination is carried out. As a routine, 1.5 cc of Conray 60 is injected. Particular attention is paid to the volume accepted and the radiologic configuration of the contrast. A normal disc rarely accepts more than 0.75 cc.

In order to avoid the risk of a high volume

of contrast material which may neutralize chymopapain, a period of 15 minutes is allowed to lapse before injecting the enzyme. As previously stated, chymopapain is very thermolabile and should be removed from the refrigerator and reconstituted immediately before injection. Four thousand units (4000) of chymopapain is injected per disc and the amount used should not exceed ten thousand (10,000) per patient. After 15 minutes, when the risk of an anaphylactic reaction has passed, the administration of the anesthetic is discontinued, the patient is extubated and transferred to the recovery room.

POSTOPERATIVE CARE

After chemonucleolysis, all patients experience low back discomfort which may require the administration of narcotic analgesics for at least the first 24 hours. Ambulation is begun within 12–36 hours depending on the patient's clinical status. The average stay in the hospital after chemonucleolysis is 3 days. The postchemonucleolysis course is quite variable. The amount of back pain is not predictable and has no relation to age of the patient, the duration of symptoms, or the number of discs injected. Patients are treated symptomatically with anti-inflammatory medication, analgesics, and muscle relaxants. Corsets are not prescribed routinely. Occasionally, a patient may develop a list of the spine which requires a Camp corset or chair-back type brace for several weeks.

It is extremely important to emphasize to the patient that he has undergone an operation and a healing period is necessary. To minimize the morbidity after the procedure, patients are advised to restrict sitting for the first 4–6 weeks during the period of settling of the treated disc spaces. The time required to return to regular activities varies. White collar personnel should be allowed 4–12 weeks off from work; blue collar or manual workers require 3–6 months before returning to their duties.

Patients are routinely seen for the first time in follow-up 6 weeks after chemonucleolysis. Unusual pain or temperature elevation logically would prompt an earlier evaluation. Clinical and radiologic assessment is carried out during the return visit. Narrowing of the treated disc spaces is expected, with maximum narrowing being attained 3 months postchemonucleolysis. The final clinical assessment is made 6 months after the procedure.

RESULTS

Since 1973, the author has treated approximately 600 patients, using the technique described previously. Between 1973 and 1980, 373 patients were treated and 345 of these were re-examined or answered a detailed questionnaire. The minimum follow-up period was 1 year and some of the cases were followed up to 8.5 years.

The results were classified according to Macnab's criteria.[29] Excellent or good results were considered satisfactory, while fair or poor results were rated as unsatisfactory. Satisfactory results were obtained in 77% of cases. In procedures carried out after 1975, excluding previously operated cases and workmen's compensation cases, satisfactory results were obtained in 88%. Table 9.1 details the number of levels injected in relation to the grading of the results obtained.

COMPLICATIONS

In this series of 373 patients, a severe anaphylactic reaction occurred in two

Table 9.1. Number of levels injected and results obtained

Levels Injected	Ratio of Satisfactory/Total	Satisfactory Rate
L3–4	6/8	75%
L4–5	47/59	80%
L5–S1	67/80	84%
2-level	117/160	73%
3-level	25/32	78%
4-level	5/6	83%

cases. Both cases were successfully managed by the attending anaesthesiologist. There were five minor delayed sensitivity reactions without adverse consequences. Discitis occurred in one case and was treated successfully by antibiotic therapy with complete recovery.

Watts[30] published a detailed report of the first 13,700 patients who underwent chemonucleolysis. The complication rate in this series was 2.9%, a rate considerably less than complication rate reported by Spangfort[31] after open surgery.

A few other possible complications related to the procedure should be mentioned, all of which can be avoided if proper precautions are taken. Positioning of the patient in the lateral decubitus position should be done with care to avoid an upper extremity nerve palsy. Cushioning of the knee is important to prevent a peroneal nerve palsy.

The possibility of injuring a nerve root exists, particularly at the L5-S1 disc level, if the needle is not inserted properly. The author has not seen progression of a neurologic deficit nor sciatica attributable to nerve root injury. If the needle is advanced slowly, the nerve root will move when touched by the needle tip. If the leg should twitch when the tip is advanced, the needle should be withdrawn. Multiple attempts at entering the L5-S1 space from the lateral approach should be discontinued. The operator then should resort to the posterior transdural discographic approach in such an instance.

FAILURES OF CHEMONUCLEOLYSIS

In spite of the excellent results obtained, possible causes of failure should be considered carefully.

(1) Enzyme instability. In three patients, symptomatic relief did not occur and no disc narrowing was observed 6 weeks after chemonucleolysis. At the time of surgical intervention in these cases, disc herniations were seen and the nucleus pulposus was removed. It must be assumed that the chymopapain was inactive at the time of the injection of the enzyme.

It is extremely important to stress that proper refrigeration must be maintained during delivery and storage of chymopapain. Reconstitution of the enzyme should be carried out immediately before injection.

(2) Lumbar instability. Preoperatively, it is difficult to identify with absolute accuracy the patient needing a fusion at the time of discectomy. Two schools of thought exist in that respect.[32] One school believes that all patients who undergo discectomy should have a fusion performed at that level at the same time. The second school proposes staging of the surgical procedure, suggesting initial discectomy be followed by fusion if back pain persists. The current trend favors the latter approach.[33]

It has been the author's experience that after chemonucleolysis, the need for surgical stabilization is considerably less than by discectomy. The normal tissue surrounding the disc is not injured in the process of chemonucleolysis, whereas it is violated in the process of a surgical intervention.

CONCLUDING COMMENTS

The central fact which can be deduced from this clinical experience is that chemonucleolysis is an effective procedure in the management of lumbar disc herniations in properly selected cases. In countries where the use of the enzyme is not restricted, one finds enthusiastic proponents. Successful results have been reported that are comparable to the best results obtained by surgical intervention. It has been the author's experience that the risk of anaphylaxis is far less than the complications which may be incurred after an operative intervention.

Discectomy should be reserved for those cases in which chemonucleolysis is not successful. In a certain number of patients, symptomatic relief of sciatica will be observed after disc dissolution though back pain will increase. This type of patient represents the group which may require a lumbar fusion because of an underlying instability problem.

A fear frequently voiced is that chymopapain may leak out from the nucleus pulposus or enter the blood circulation. Within seconds of injecting the enzyme intradiscally, it becomes irreversibly bound to the substrate, and active enzyme cannot be recovered.[34] A second line of defense is provided by the α-2 macroglobulins in plasma and cerebrospinal fluid.[34] These substances are general inhibitors of proteolytic enzymes. It should be stated that although leakage is a possibility, for practical reasons, the danger is minimal.

Chemonucleolysis has been slow to achieve universal popularity. It is obviously not a panacea for all lumbosacral disorders, although it is effective in the management of back pain and sciatica caused by herniation of the nucleus pulposus. Chemonucleolysis requires the surgeon to establish firmly the proper diagnosis before instituting this form of therapy. With proper patient selection, it should be expected that good results can be obtained in the majority of patients.

References

1. Mixter, W. J., Barr, J. S.: Rupture of the intervertebral disc with involvement of the spinal canal. *N. Engl. J. Med. 211:*210, 1934.
2. Lindbloom, K.: Diagnostic puncture of intervertebral discs in sciatica. *Acta Orthop. Scand. 17:*231, 1948.
3. Hirsch, C.: Studies on the pathology of low back pain. *J. Bone Joint Surg. 41B:*237–243, 1959.
4. Smith, L., Garvin, P. Q., Gesher, R. M., et al: Enzyme dissolution of the nucleus pulposus. *Nature (London) 198:*1311–1312, 1963.
5. Smith, L.: Enzyme dissolution of the nucleus pulposus in humans. *J.A.M.A. 187:*137–140, 1964.
6. Stern, I.: Chemonucleolysis seminar sponsored by Flint Laboratories of Canada, Montreal, November 19, 1977.
7. Garvin, P. J., Jennings, R. B., Smith, L., Gesler, R. M.: Chymopapain—a pharmacological and toxicological evaluation in experimental animals. *Clin. Orthop. 42:*204, 223, 1965.
8. Garvin, P. J., Jennings, R. B., Stern, I. J.: Enzymatic digestion of the nucleus pulposus: A review

of experimental studies with chymopapain. *Orthop. Clin. North Am. 8(1):*27–35, January 1977.
9. Shealy, C. N.: Tissue reaction to chymopapain in cats. *J. Neurosurg. 26(3):*327, 1967.
10. Rydevik, B., Branemark, P. T., Nordberg, C., McLean, W. G., Sjostrand, J., Fogelberg, M.: Effects of chymopapain on nerve tissue. *Spine 1:*137, 1976.
11. Macnab, I., McCulloch, J. A., Weiner, D. S., Hugo, E. P., Galway, R. D., Dall, D.: Chemonucleolysis. *Canad. J. Surg. 14(4):*280, 1971.
12. Ford, L. T.: Experimental study of chymopapain in cats. *Clin. Orthop. 67:*68, 1969.
13. Macnab, I., McCulloch, J. A., Weiner, D. S., Hugo, E. P., Galway, R. D., Dall, D.: Chemonucleolysis. *Canad. J. Surg. 14(4):*280, 1971.
14. Garvin, P. J., Jennings, R. B., Stern, I. J.: Enzymatic digestion of the nucleus pulposus: A review of experimental studies with chymopapain. *Orthop. Clin. North Am. 8(1):*27–35, January 1977.
15. Stern, I. J., Smith, L.: Dissolution by chymopapain in vitro of tissue from normal or prolapsed intervertebral discs. *Clin. Orthop. 50:*269, 1967.
16. Stern, I. J., Cosmas, F., Smith, L.: Urinary polyuronide excretion in man after enzymatic dissolution of the chondromucoprotein of the intervertebral disc or surgical stress. *Clin. Chim. Acta 21:*181–190, 1968.
17. Hendry, N. G. C.: The hydration of the nucleus pulposus and its relation to intervertebral disc degeneration. *J. Bone Joint Surg. 40B:*132–144, 1958.
18. Naylor, A., Smare, D. L.: Fluid content of the nucleuc pulposus as a factor in the disc syndrome. *Br. Med. J. 2:*975–976, 1953.
19. Sutton, J. C. in publication.
20. Day, P. L.: Early, interim and long term observations on chemonucleolysis in 876 patients with special comments on the lateral approach. *Clin. Orthop. 99:*64–49, 1974.
21. Javid, M. J.: Treatment of herniated lumbar disc syndrome with chymopapain. *J.A.M.A. 243(20):*2043–48, 1980.
22. Bradford, D., Garcia, A.: Herniations of the lumbar intervertebral disc in children and adolescents. A review of thirty surgically treated cases. *J.A.M.A. 210:*2045, 1969.
23. Key, J.: Intervertebral disc lesions in children and adolescents. *J. Bone Joint Surg. 32A:*97, 1950.
24. McCulloch, J. A.: Chemonucleolysis: Experience with 2000 cases. *Clin. Orthop. 146:*128–135, 1980.
25. Day, P. L.: Sicot, Symposium on Chemonucleolysis. Israel, October 9–13, 1972.
26. Hashimoto, K., Hashimoto, K.: The mechanism of sensitization of the ventricle to epinephrine by halothane. *Am. Heart J. 83:*652–658, 1972.
27. Katz, R. L., Epstein, R. A.: The interaction of anesthetic agents and adrenergic drugs to produce cardiac arrhythmias. *Anesthesiology 29:*763–784, 1968.
28. Mathews, K. P.: Adverse reactions to drugs; Hypersensitivity. In: *Current Therapy*, W. B. Saunders, Philadelphia, Conn, H. F. (Ed). 1981, p. 647–653.

29. MacNab, I.: Negative disc exploration. *J. Bone Joint Surg. 53A:*891, 1971.
30. Watts, C.: Complications of chemonucleolysis for lumbar disc disease. *Neurosurgery 1:*2–5, 1977.
31. Spangfort, E. V.: The lumbar disc herniation. A computer-aided analysis of 2,504 operations. *Acta Orthop. Scand. 142 (suppl):*1–95, 1972.
32. Farfan, H. F.: Personal communication.
33. Wiltse, L. L.: Surgery for intervertebral disc disease of the lumbar spine. *Clin. Orthop. 129:*22, 1977.
34. Barrett, A. J., Starkey, P. M.: The interaction of alpha-2-macroglobulin with proteinases. *Biochem. J. 133:*709–724, 1973.

10

The Diagnosis and Treatment of Spinal Infections

Vertebral infections encompassing both intervertebral disc space infection and vertebral osteomyelitis present a varied and difficult challenge, not only in diagnosis but also in antimicrobial and surgical treatment.

The special anatomical considerations involving the spine and disc space present problems. The lack of tissue penetration of antibiotics and the type of surgery that is performed for herniated nucleus pulposus can predispose the patient to the development of postoperative infections in a closed space. These aspects, and particularly the selection of antimicrobial agents and new developments surrounding their use, will be discussed.

DISCITIS

Intervertebral disc space infection, "discitis," is defined as an inflammatory and presumably infectious involvement of the intervertebral disc. The symptoms are different in the child and the adult. In the child, it may be difficult to elicit various symptoms. The child may present only as a fussy, crying individual who finds it difficult to sit or ambulate, indicating pain in the low back. Indeed, the failure of a child to maintain a previously normal posture without pain may be a cardinal sign of the disease. At the time that the child is experiencing this presentation, he may have accompanying fever and chills. Nonspecific symptoms such as malaise, poor appetite, and disinterest also may be present. If the process is located above the level of T10,

there is usually less pain in both the child and the adult due to decreased movement of the spine in this area. Below this level, the general weight-bearing stress produces significant pain. A careful examination usually will reveal tenderness to percussion over the affected vertebra; this is usually one of the important signs on physical examination. The laboratory may or may not show significant abnormalities in the blood count. After a certain period of time, a nonspecific anemia usually appears. Leukocytosis is not always present, especially at the outset. Invariably, by the time the patient seeks attention, the erythrocyte sedimentation rate is elevated. Calcium, phosphorus, and alkaline phosphatase levels are generally not helpful. Serum alkaline phosphatase in the child is usually elevated due to growth. Blood cultures, if positive, are the single most helpful tests. Too frequently, when the process is detected, the bacteremia, if due to hematogenous spread to the lumbar spine, has since ended. A positive blood culture, however, allows isolation of the etiologic organism obviating the need to perform an invasive procedure to obtain the organism. If the blood cultures are negative and there is radiographic clinical evidence of a diseased vertebra or disc, some authorities recommend aspiration with proper radiographic guidance.[1] The isolation of the etiologic bacterial agent is most important since any organism has been shown to cause osteomyelitis and discitis. Most common, however, is staphylococcus, especially in the young child. In the adult, the staphylococus or a gram-negative organism originating from the gastrointestinal or urinary tract becomes more prevalent

The most useful diagnostic tool, early in the course of the disease when x-rays are invariably negative, is the bone scan[2] (Fig. 10.1). Early, this is positive due to the hyperemia about the area with the inflammatory response. Later it is positive due to the actual involvement of the bone itself (Figs. 10.2 and 10.3).

There is a growing consensus that discitis should be considered infectious in origin despite reports of cures obtained solely by immobilization and without the use of any systemic antimicrobial therapy.[3-5] To explain this, one has to observe the difference in blood supply to the intervertebral disc space in the child versus the adult.[6] The vascular supply decreases significantly with age and successful treatment of a child by immobilization is probably related to the recuperative abilities of a young patient[7] (Figs. 10.4 and 10.5). The concept of a "sterile" inflammatory discitis is fallacious.

The initial choice of an antibiotic can be best assisted by examining a Gram stain of aspirated material, pending a culture. The fact that anaerobic, as well as microaerophilic organisms can attack the spine and produce the disease should influence the physician to make appropriate arrangements with the laboratory for suitable culturing in special media. Special types of patients are more prone to different etiologic organisms. Diabetics and heroin addicts more commonly have a staphylococcal or pseudomonas infection. Elderly patients, especially males, with chronic or recurrent urinary tract infections will commonly have a gram-negative enteric infection.[8, 9] Young, otherwise healthy individuals usually harbor a staphylococcus infection[10] (Table 10.1).

Rarely, one is surprised by a very odd organism in a patient without an obvious cause (Figs. 10.6 and 10.7). This usually makes isolation of the organism essential, a technique which can significantly lessen

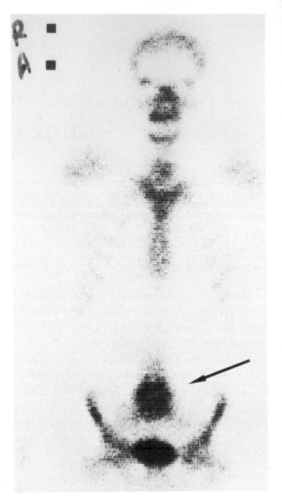

Figure 10.1. Bone scan in patient with a postoperative disc space infection.

morbidity by the proper initial choice of an antibiotic.

OSTEOMYELITIS

Much of what has been said concerning the diagnosis and isolation of the bacterial agent in discitis also applies to osteomyelitis. Osteomyelitis *de novo* does not have to be associated with accompanying discitis. The use of the bone scan is the premier tool of diagnosis. "Cold" bone scans, however, have been described in acute osteomyelitis due presumably to local ischemia secondary to a subperiosteal collection of pus.[11] A

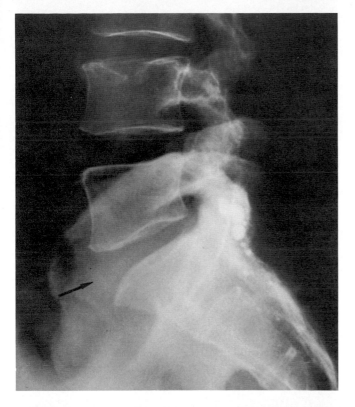

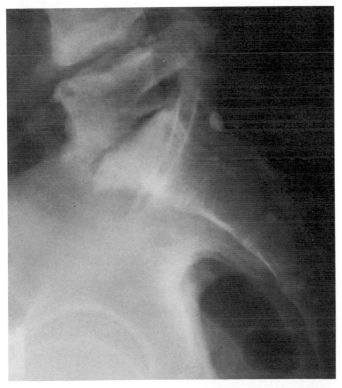

Figures 10.2 and 10.3. Sequence of lumbar spine x-rays showing infection before and after L5-S1 postoperative disc space infection. Note narrowing of space.

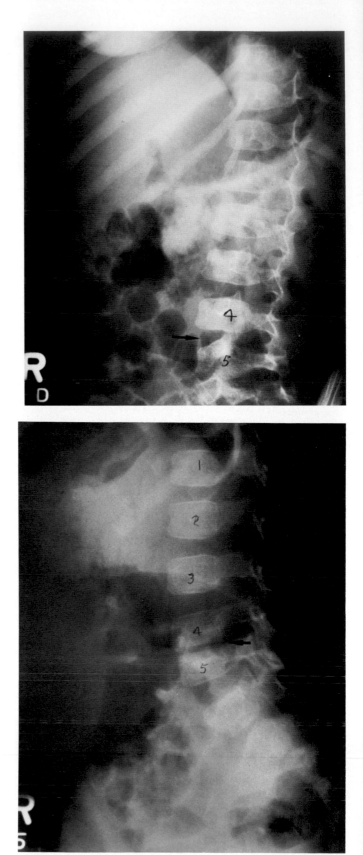

Figures 10.4 and 10.5. Discitis is shown in a 3-year-old child with narrowing of the disc space, L4–5. No etiologic organism isolated.

Table 10.1. The association between prodromal infection and infections of the intervertebral disc is shown

Case number	Primary infection and complications	Organism isolated from primary infections	Pre-operative antibiotic in therapeutic dosage	Organism isolated from disc at operation
1	Pyelitis	B. proteus (urine)	No	B. proteus
2	Enlarged prostate: self-instrumentation knitting needle	E. coli: B. proteus (urine)	No	E. coli
3	Chronic dermatitis. Secondarily infected	Staph. pyogenes (skin)	No	Staph. pyogenes
4	Rh.A. (10 years). Pyogenic polyarthritis (2 years previously). Recurrent furunculosis	Staph. pyogenes (furuncle)	No	E. coli: B. proteus
7	No known infection	Negative	No	B. proteus
8	Nephrolithotomy. Recurrent pyelitis, Diabetes Mellitus (D.M.)	E. coli (urine)	Yes	Negative
9	Herpes zoster. Secondarily infected	Negative	No	Negative
10	No known infection	Negative	No	Staph. pyogenes
12	Recurrent pyelitis (D.M. 10 years)	E. coli (urine)	Yes	Negative
13	Phlebitis. Septicaemia. Septic broncho-pneumonia	Staph. pyogenes (blood, urine, sputum)	No	Staph. pyogenes
14	Otitis media. Bronchopleural fistula. Septic bronchopneumonia (D.M.)	Strep. pneumoniae (sputum). Staph. pyogenes (sputum)	Yes	Staph. pyogenes
15	Known drug addict. ? Intravenous administration	Negative	No	Staph. pyogenes

gallium scan has been helpful in some of these cases.[12]

Complications of osteomyelitis include the following: (1) paraplegia—this is a dreaded complication where the mechanism usually is scarring with traction on the nerves and associated septic thrombosis of the spinal vessels; (2) epidural (extradural) abscess—this usually is seen as a direct extension of the primary infection; (3) cerebrospinal fluid extension resulting in meningitis—this usually is due to penetration of the dura with perforation and spread of the infection throughout the cerebrospinal fluid. These complications are best avoided by prompt diagnosis and therapy with the use of adjunctive surgical therapy to decompress and drain a mass lesion. Once extension into the cerebrospinal fluid results, a true medical emergency exists.

The predilection, especially in the adult, for hematogenous spread to the bones is due to the development of a rich intraosseous vertebral body venous plexus. In the intervertebral disc, the blood supply decreases with advancing age. In the vertebral body, blood supply increases. There can be involvement of more than one body due to the freely anastomosing channels of two adjacent vertebral bodies. Another anatomical anomaly that predisposes to this problem is that of the extension from the pelvis due to avalvular venous anastomosis described by Batson.[13]

ANTIMICROBIAL THERAPY IN SPINAL INFECTIONS

A general rule in the treatment of bacterial infections is to use the best agent, pref-

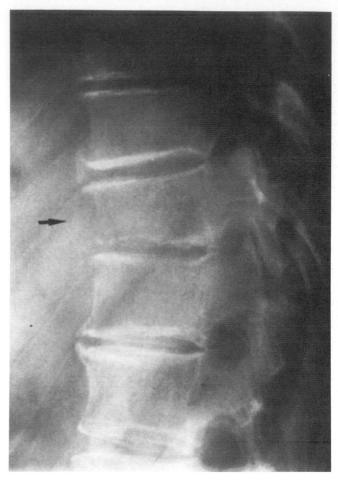

Figures 10.6 and 10.7. Vertebral osteomyelitis (adult) progression of changes is shown. Organism is *Hemophilus aphrophilus*.

erably bacteriocidal, that penetrates into the infected tissues. At the outset, an antibiotic should always be administered parenterally for these types of infections. The concentration of the agent in the blood should be monitored and, preferably, an organism obtained by culture, allowing determination of its susceptibility.

This is done by several microbiological techniques: (1) the Kirby-Bauer disc sensitivity method;[14, 15] (2) the tube dilution minimal inhibitory concentration;[16, 17] and (3) the Schlichter test, which represents the serum dilution test against the isolated organism.[18]

Obviously, antibiotic data from past experience at a specific hospital can give a clue to the probable sensitivity of certain organisms, but some generalizations concerning treatment can be made. If a staphylococcal infection is presumed, a semisynthetic penicillinase resistant penicillin or cephalosporin agent should be used initially. If the organism is shown to be sensitive to penicillin G, then this agent should be substituted for the semisynthetic penicillin or cephalosporin. The dosage of these antibiotics should be quite high—in the range of 10–20 million units of penicillin G, or 10 to 12 gm, or greater, for a semisynthetic penicillin or cephalosporin agent. The treatment time can be individualized but generally high dosage treatment for at least 3–4 weeks is used. Depending upon the extent of the disease and any complications, treatment should continue for at

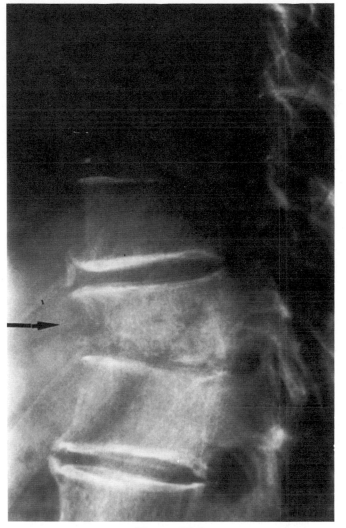

Figure 10.7.

least another month with a suitable oral agent. The addition of concomitant probenecid will allow higher blood levels due to the blocking of the drug at the distal tubule of the kidney. This drug is usually given in a dosage of 0.5 gm, 2–4 times a day, with the antibiotic.

PENICILLIN ALLERGY

If an anaphylactic reaction or serious documented penicillin reaction has occurred in the past, prudence would dictate not using this agent unless adequate skin testing is done first. This usually poses a problem since the patient has to be treated quickly. Testing with a minor determinant mixture and the use of a penicilloyl polylysine (PPL) skin test should be performed.[19, 20] If there is a significant reaction to either of these agents, a penicillin agent should not be given. If the skin test is negative, a penicillin and/or cephalosporin agent to which there is some cross-sensitivity should be given very cautiously. In such cases where clear-cut anaphylactic reaction exists, vancomycin can be employed. This agent should be given intravenously, 500

Table 10.2. Penetration of antibiotics into brain is shown

ANTIBIOTIC	AVERAGE BLOOD LEVELS (μg/ml)	AVERAGE BRAIN LEVELS (μg/gm)	BLOOD/BRAIN RATIO
Chloramphenicol	4.0	36.0	1/9
Cephalothin	11.7	1.6	7/1
Ampicillin	21.3	0.4	56/1
Penicillin	7.5	0.32	23/1
Cephaloridine	18.04	0.90	20/1

After Kramer PW, Griffith RS, Campbell RL: Antibiotic penetration of the brain. A comparative study. J Neurosurg *31*:300, 1969 Table 2.

mg every 6 hours for a total dose of 2 gm in a 24-hour period. This should never be given by bolus injection, but should rather be allowed to infuse over a 60-minute period of time. This agent, however, has no significant penetration into the cerebrospinal fluid and should not be used when meningitis is suspected.

Gram-negative spinal or meningeal infection also can be treated with an aminoglycoside (gentamicin, tobromycin, amikacin). It must be given intrathecally for meningitis or ventriculitis.[21]

Two very recently released third generation cephalosporins, cefotaxime and moxalactam, show penetration into the cerebrospinal fluid when used in high dose (12–16 gm, daily).[22, 23]

If involvement of the meninges or neural tissue is suspected, chloramphenicol could be employed (Table 10.2). A word of caution regarding chloramphenicol is in order. This drug should never be used prophylactically when another antibiotic with similar tissue penetration is available. A severe unpredictable hypersensitivity bone marrow reaction may occur in as many as 1 in 20,000 administrations. This is irreversible even when the dosage is decreased or the drug is discontinued. Careful observation of serial blood counts will not predict development of a fatal, irreversible aplastic bone marrow reaction, but will help in preventing dosage-related reversible bone marrow suppression. Penetration into the brain, as well as the meninges, with chloramphenicol is greater than with any other antibiotic. The brain-to-serum ratio is the highest obtainable.

Recently anaerobic infections due to sensitive organisms have responded well to metronidazole, 2 gm daily in four divided doses. This drug penetrates very well into the brain and meninges.

In a gram-negative aerobic infection, isolation of the organism is important due to a growing resistance which is transferable via plasmid-mediated resistance factors.[24] Bacteriocidal antibiotics, either an aminoglycoside or cephalosporin in appropriate doses to achieve adequate serum and tissue levels, should be chosen. Monitoring for aminoglycoside therapy generally is now available with results within 24 hours or less. A serum trough and peak level should be obtained just prior to and 1 hour after a dose of the agent. Toxic and therapeutic levels are determined for each laboratory and technique employed.

PROPHYLAXIS

The mechanisms involving the growth of organisms in a surgical wound are elucidated poorly. Obviously, surgical technique and attention to the integrity of blood supply and diminution of tissue trauma are most important. It has been shown that 20 minutes after rendering the skin sterile with preoperative bactericidal agents and scrub-

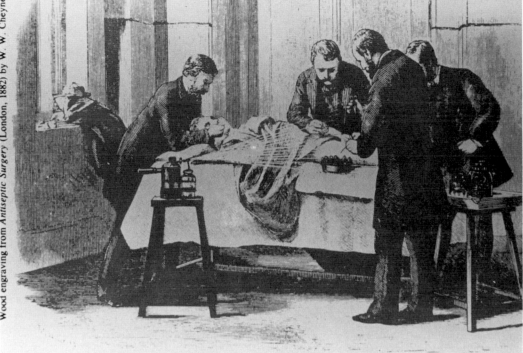

A Lister carbolic spray provides antiseptic protection during an operation.

Figure 10.8. Attempt at antiseptic environment during surgery using a Lister carbolic spray is shown (woodcut).

bing, organisms may inhabit the area. The size of the inoculum, as well as certain agents, predispose the patient to a wound infection (Fig. 10.8).

Wound infections are generally of two types: the immediate, most often occurring in the hospital or shortly after discharge, which usually brings the patient back to the hospital, and the late, which is usually encountered after the wound is well-healed. This is probably the result of a latent infection which has been suppressed by the use of perioperative prophylactic antibiotics. This practice may allow the organism to remain viable but inactive until certain conditions allow it to become more active and cause a clinical infection. The widespread use of prophylactic antibiotics in clean surgery has been documented to be associated with an increase in resistant organisms found on certain hospital units. A British study in a neurosurgical unit producing resistant Klebsiella infection was due to the widespread use of prophylactic antibiotics in clean cases.[25]

Local prophylaxis of the wound at the time of surgery has been in existence for some time. The Mt. Sinai regimen consists of gentamicin (80 mg intravenously), vancomycin (1 gm intravenously) and local irrigant saline solution consisting of streptomycin (50 mg/liter).[26] This regimen results in good soft tissue, skin, bone, and muscle concentration of antibiotics but no appreciable cerebrospinal fluid or central nervous system penetration. The use of special equipment such as laminar flow operating rooms or a portable unit has not been shown to be of consistent benefit to be cost effective.

Wood engraving from *Antiseptic Surgery* (London, 1882) by W. W. Cheyne

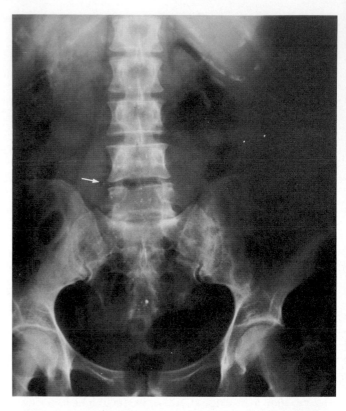

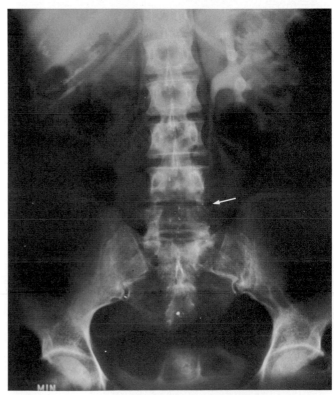

Figures 10.9–10.11. X-rays showing L4–5 postoperative disc space infection. Note narrowing of disc space and sclerosis and bridging of the intervertebral disc space.

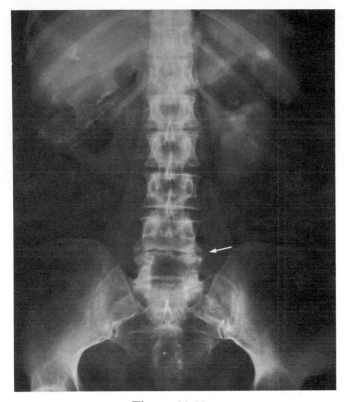

Figure 10.11.

POSTOPERATIVE SPINAL INFECTIONS

The dramatic recurrence of severe back pain 1–6 weeks postoperatively should alert the clinician to the possibility of operative site infection. The temperature may or may not be elevated. Initially, no radiologic changes are noted. Subsequently, a sequence of events with loss of height of the disc space, irregular destruction of the end plates and eventual sclerosis is seen (Figs. 10.9–10.11). As in the nonoperative infections, etiologic diagnosis should be confirmed by aspiration or operative means. This is important in that the patient may have an operative space abscess formation at this area requiring incision and drainage.[27] A dread complication of a postoperative wound infection is penetration into the cerebropsinal fluid, as well as a toxic syndrome resulting from a septicemia.

SUMMARY

The concept of juvenile discitis as a sterile inflammatory disease should be abandoned. Aggressive attempts to produce an etiologic agent in both osteomyelitis and in discitis should be made.

The use of the bone scan early in the course of the disease is recommended, especially when the radiograph is negative. Computerized axial tomography scan should be employed if any doubt exists or if the bone scan is questionable (Fig. 10.12).

The proper use of antibiotics, initially using a bacteriocidal agent that will penetrate into the site of the infection, with proper monitoring based upon sensitivity tests and serum concentration, is mandatory.

A high index of suspicion, alerting the physician to a postoperative wound infection, should be maintained in any patient

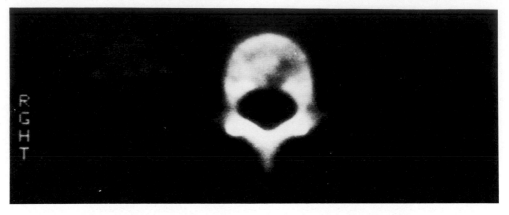

Figure 10.12. Computerized axial tomography shows osteomyelitis of the lumbar vertebra in a 3-year-old child.

who becomes febrile and begins having symptoms after initially doing well postoperatively.

Finally, there has been little success in selecting a prophylactic regimen. No local, systemic, or combination regimen has been found effective in prevention of infections in the postoperative state. Emergence of organisms resistant to antimicrobial agents will continue to be a problem. An ongoing search for new antibiotic agents which will keep pace with evolving modes of genetic resistance patterns is mandatory.

References

1. Wenger, D. R., Bobechko, W. P., Gilday, D. L.: The spectrum of intervertebral disc space infection in children. *J. Bone Joint Surg. 60A*:100–108, 1978.
2. Rosenthal, L.: The role of strontium-85 in detection of bone disease. *Radiology 84*:75–82, 1965.
3. Kemp, H. B. S., Jackson, J. W., Jeremiah, J. D., Hall, A. J.: Acute discitis. *J. Bone Joint Surg. 54B*:753, 1972.
4. Jordan, M. C., Kirby, W. M.: Pyogenic vertebral osteomyelitis. *Arch. Intern. Med. 128*:405–410, 1971.
5. Dich, V., Nelson, J., Hultalin, K.: Osteomyelitis in infants and children. *Am. J. Dis. Child. 129*:1273–1278, 1975.
6. Waldvogel, R., Medoff, G., Swartz, M.: Osteomyelitis: A review of clinical features, therapeutic considerations, and unusual aspects. *New Engl. J. Med. 282*:316–322, 1970.
7. Taylor, T. K. F., Grainger, W. D.: Disc space infection as a complication of disc surgery. *J. Bone Joint Surg. 55B*:435, 1973.
8. Griffiths, H. E. D., Jones, D. M.: Pyogenic infec-

tion of the spine. *J. Bone Joint Surg. 53B*:383–391, 1971.
9. Winters, J. L., Cohen, I.: Acute hematogenous osteomyelitis: A review of 66 cases. *J. Bone Joint Surg. 42A*:691–704, 1960.
10. Stone, D. B., Bonfiglio, M.: Pyogenic vertebral osteomyelitis: A diagnostic pitfall for the internist. *Arch. Intern. Med. 112*:491–500, 1963.
11. Jones, D. C., Cady, R. B.: "Cold" bone scans in acute osteomyelitis. *J. Bone Joint Surg. 63B*:376–378, 1981.
12. Teates, C. D., Williamson, B. R. J.: "Hot and cold" bone lesions in acute osteomyelitis. *Am. J. Radiol. 127*:511–518, 1977.
13. Batson, O. V.: The function of the vertebral veins and their role in the spread of metastases. *Ann. Surg. 112*:138–149, 1940.
14. Bauer, A. W., Kirby, W. M., Sherris, J. C., Turck, M.: Antibiotic susceptibility testing by a standardized single disc method. *Am. J. Clin. Pathol. 45*:493–496, 1966.
15. *Federal Register. Rules and Regulations.* Antibiotic Susceptibility Discs. 37: 20525–20529, 1972.
16. Petersdorf, R. G., Plorde, J. J.: The usefulness of *in vitro* sensitivity tests in antibiotics therapy. *Ann. Rev. Med. 14*:41–56, 1963.
17. Dunlap, S. G.: The serum dilution bactericidal test for antibiotic effectiveness. *Am. J. Med. Technol. 31*:69–76, 1965.
18. Schlichter, J. G., Mclean, H.: A method of determining the effective therapeutic level in the treatment of subacute bacterial endocarditis with penicillin. *Am. Heart J. 34*:209–211, 1947.
19. Levine, B. B.: Studies on the mechanism of the formation of the penicillin antigen. *J. Exptl. Med. 112*:1131–1156, 1960.
20. Parker, C. W.: Drug allergy. *N. Engl. J. Med. 292*:951–960, 1975.
21. Mangi, R. J., Holstein, L. L., Andriole, V. T.: Treatment of gram-negative bacillary meningitis with intrathecal gentamicin. *Yale J. Biol. Med. 50*:31, 1977.
22. Schaad, U. B., McCracken, G. H. Jr., Loock, C. A., Thomas, M. L.: Pharmakokinetics and bacterio-

logic efficacy of moxalactam, cefotoxime, cefoperazone and rochephin in experimental meningitis. *J. Infect. Dis.* 143:156–163, 1981.

23. Landesman, S. H., Shah, P. M., Armengand, M., Barza, M., Cherubin, C. E.: Past and current roles of cephalosporin antibiotics in treatment of meningitis. *Am. J. Med.* 71:693–703, 1981.

24. Watanabe, T.: The origin of R factors. *Ann. N. Y. Acad. Sci.* 182:126–140, 1971.

25. Price, D. J. E., Sleigh, J. D.: Control of infection due to Klebsiella aerogenes in a neurosurgical unit by withdrawal of all antibiotics. *Lancet* 2:1213–1215, 1970.

26. Savitz, M. H.: The use of prophylactic antibiotics in neurosurgery. Chapter in: *Current Controversies in Neurosurgery*, Morley, T. P. (Ed). pp. 648–650, 1976.

27. Thibodeau, A. A.: Closed space infection following removal of lumbar intervertebral disc. *J. Bone Joint Surg.* 50A:400–410, 1968.

11

The Etiology of the "Failed Back Surgery Syndrome"*

The "failed back surgery syndrome" (FBSS) (the failure of lumbar spine surgery to relieve pain and incapacitation) is unfortunately a common phenomenon in our present society. This entity is one of the most difficult therapeutic challenges to medicine because it represents a complex interplay of organic, psychologic, and socioeconomic factors. FBSS patients *can* be "salvaged" by skilled comprehensive rehabilitation effort and can be returned to a reasonable functional status. It is eminently more reasonable, however, on the basis of what is presently known regarding FBSS, to endeavor to *prevent* it. FBSS is not only a failure of medical care but also represents, in terms of medical care costs and lost worker productivity, one of the greatest finanical losses known in the health care field.

In 1981, the total health care cost in the United States was estimated by Arthur D. Little, Inc. to be $235 billion.[1] Tobias[2] has recently determined that, in the same year, workers' compensation health care costs accounted for $25 billion of the total. Our studies show that while low back pain represents 30% of workers' compensation claims, it actually accounts for about 60% of all monies spent. The remarkable past ineffectiveness of low back care is attested to by the legions of FBSS patients who represent about 25% of all patients undergoing back surgery. It is not unusual for an insurance carrier to have escrowed as much as $1,000,000 to cover the potential costs for a FBSS patient.[3]

The author has reviewed 100 consecutive FBSS patients treated in 1974 and compared them to a group in 1981. The "typical" patient in the 1974 group was middle-aged and had undergone 3.6 low back operations and 2.8 iophendylate myelograms at the time of the initial interview. By 1981, the average number of previous surgeries per referred FBSS patient had decreased to 1.96. In the typical case, the historic review suggested that the initial back problem was either a posterior nerve root irritation syndrome (disc bulge or mechanical type pain) or an anterior nerve root irritation/compression syndrome (disc herniation compressing spinal nerve or lateral spinal stenosis). These syndromes are explained more fully later in this chapter.

Back pain frequently was associated with a sciatic radiculitis characterized by pain radiating to the feet or toes, accompanied by nerve tenderness to palpation at the sciatic notch and popliteal fossa. Positive straight leg raising was commonly present, as were reflex or sensory changes. Motor deficits were uncommon.

* The author would like to express his appreciation to his associates: Charles Ray, M.D., Alex Lifson, M.D., Kenneth Heithoff, M.D., Harvey Aaron, M.D., and Gail Nida, R.N. for their professional support and encouragement, and to Mary Anne Wilson, R.N., Mary Carroll, R.N., Barbara Deede, R.N., Kevin Gracie, Lois Bredeson, Darla Becker, Paula Kraay, and Kay Robertson for their clinical support and assistance in preparing this paper.

The entire medical staff at our Institute extends to William Kirkaldy-Willis, M.D. our appreciation and sincere thanks. His leadership and dedicated teaching is largely responsible for the advances in applied clinical sciences described here.

The Minnesota Multiphasic Personality Inventory test (MMPI) is routinely used for patient evaluation, and is expected to show elevation of the hysteria, hypchondriasis, and depression scales. FBSS patients with a "normal" profile are subject to additional scrutiny, as are individuals in whom affective disorders are present.

In FBSS, the chronic use of analgesics and narcotics depressing endogenous opiate production[4] (and thus, *increasing* pain) is common. Equally deleterious is the chronic use of muscle relaxants, which often serve to increase depression and also thereby enhance pain.

This chapter reviews the author's experience in the rehabilitation of about 3000 FBSS patients over the past 10 years. An attempt will be made to define and convey what has been learned so that this information can serve as the basis for a new approach to the low back pain problem.

The following statements summarize the basic reasons for the current large numbers of FBSS patients:

(1) There is insufficient public education regarding the back.

(2) There is a lack of risk-identification and preventive programs in home and industry.

(3) There is insufficient effective conservative care for basic low back problems.

(4) There is inadequate diagnostic information regarding the pathologic process prior to surgery.

(5) Iatrogenically induced disease.

In 1981, *Clinical Orthopedics*[5] published the results of an interinstitutional study on the basic *organic* causes of FBSS from the Sister Kenny Institute and the University Hospital, Saskatoon (Table 11.1). From these data, it can be seen that by the appreciation of these entities it is possible to avoid or effectively treat them. It must be carefully pointed out that the chronic FBSS case represents a complex interplay of functional and organic disease, and both must be addressed. Rehabilitative effort for such patients consists of: (1) treatment of chemical abuse or dependency, (2) enhancing endogenous opiate metabolism, (3) chronic pain rehabilitation involving mental and physical reactivation, (4) identification of nerve compression and its surgical relief when appropriate, (5) avoiding the creation of additional iatrogenic disease, (6) appli-

Table 11.1. Primary factors leading to FBSS (excluding spondylolisthesis)*

Primary Factors	Sister Kenny Institute	University Hospital Saskatoon
Lateral spinal stenosis	58%	57%
Central stenosis (including fusion over growth)	7%	14%
Adhesive arachnoiditis	16%	6%
Recurrent or persistent disk herniation	12%	16%
Epidural fibrosis	8%	6%
Nerve injury during surgery	less than 5%	
Chronic mechanical pain	less than 5%	
Transitional syndrome (above fusion)	less than 5%	
Pseudoarthrosis	less than 5%	
Foreign body	less than 5%	
Surgery performed at wrong level or wrong side	less than 5%	
Unknown	less than 5%	

* This table reflects the results of FBSS patient diagnosis data collected at the Low Back Clinic of the Sister Kenny Institute and the Department of Orthopaedics at the University Hospital in Saskatoon over a 1-year period. Because the final figures are averaged, the totals do not add up to 100%. (Reprinted from *Clin. Orthop. 157:*192, 1981.)

cation of implanted neuroaugmentive electronic pain relief devices for relief of pain
secondary to permanent nerve injury.

LATERAL SPINAL STENOSIS

First described by neurosurgeon Henk
Verbiest,[6] lateral spinal stenosis has come
to be appreciated as an important, and relatively common, reason for low back and
leg pain. High-resolution computed tomographic (CT) scanning of the lumbar spine
has confirmed the observation by Kirkaldy-
Willis[5] of its presence in 57% of patients
coming to surgical discectomy. Figure 11.1
demonstrates the progressive changes
which occur when abnormal stress is directed to the disc, producing loss of disc
integrity and the production of segmental
instability. It would seem that nature's in-
tent is to stabilize the interspace by absorb-
ing the deranged disc and encouraging subperiosteal bone deposition leading to auto-
fusion. Clinically significant nerve root
compression occurs as the result of a number of factors, which include the size of the

central canal at birth, concurrent disc herniation, ligamentum flavum hypertrophy,
etc. Cases of nerve compression are probably uncommon when compared to the many
asymptomatic cases of foraminal narrowing, which stabilize spontaneously. Disc
space and foraminal narrowing are commonly seen in CT scans of older individuals.
It is in the 60- to 70-year-old group that
multilevel nerve compression producing
spondylotic caudal radiculopathy commonly is seen as a result of nature's inability
to "cope."

Figure 11.2 illustrates some of the common sites of spinal nerve and ganglion compression. At L4–5, the exiting nerve and
ganglia have been compromised by the enlarged and displaced superior articular
process of L5 and the L4 vertebrae pedicle.
This represents the entity most clinicians
think of when the term lateral spinal stenosis is used. Also shown is compression of
the S1 nerve and ganglion by a hypertrophic superior articular process of the S1
vertebrae. This is a more medial form of
lateral spinal stenosis, and the point of com-

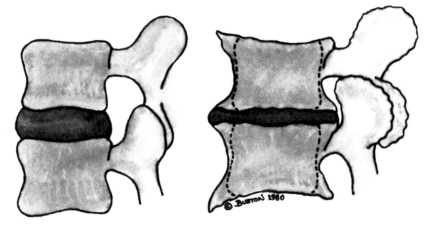

Figure 11.1. Normal and degenerative relationships: The so-called "normal" relationships are shown on the *left*. Lumbar degenerative disc disease implies the progressive loss of segmental stability. This most probably reflects normal and abnormal stress on the disc as evidenced by annular rotational strains and tears and internal disruption of the nucleus pulposus and annulus. With loss of stability, abnormal motion initiates osteoblast proliferation as evidenced by subperios-teal bone deposition, producing vertebral osteophytes and zygapophyseal hypertrophy. As these changes progress and the disc is absorbed, the intervertebral space narrows and the superior articular process of the inferior vertebrae is displaced upwards and forwards, producing stenosis of the intervertebral foramen. © Charles V. Burton, M.D.

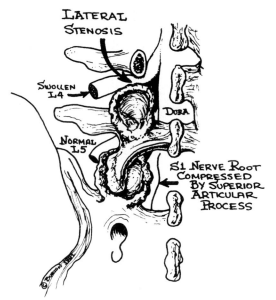

Figure 11.2. Common sites of spinal nerve and ganglion compression: The exiting L4 nerve root and ganglion has been compressed between the superior articular process of L5 and the L4 vertebral pedicle. Distal to compression the nerve is swollen. At L5-S1, the traversing S1 nerve root has been compressed in the "subarticular gutter" (or groove). It is this groove which passes along the medial border of the pedicle and leads to the intervertebral foramen. © Charles V. Burton, M.D.

promise is at the point of the subarticular "gutter" (or "groove"). Subarticular stenosis involves the *traversing* nerve root rather than the *exiting* nerve root, and the point of compression is at the "take-off" of the nerve root from the dural sac at the superior edge of the vertebrae rather than within the intervertebral foramen. In Figure 11.3, this is more clearly shown. The entity typically involves a bulging disc or annulus (not necessarily herniated) and the nerve is compressed in the course of its "rollercoaster" ride over the disc and under the articular process. I describe this as a "Guillotine phenomenon." The nerve, as shown in Figure 11.4, may be markedly distorted by the chronic pressure upon it.

When stenosis cases are accurately diagnosed, they are occasionally amenable to conservative measures but, invariably, are relieved by appropriate surgical management. It is an unfortunate fact that the commonly employed diagnostic studies, plain films and myelography, are technically incapable of providing meaningful objective diagnostic information regarding these stenosis entities. When a medial defect is seen on myelography it is invariably attributed to "disc herniation." With the

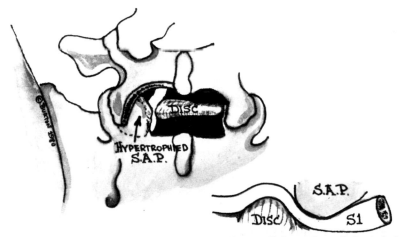

Figure 11.3. Superior articular facet compression: The medial portion of the inferior articular process of L5 has been removed to show how the traversing S1 nerve root and ganglion has been impinged under the superior articular process (*S.A.P.*) of S1. The presence of a disc or annulus bulge is often the key factor in promoting a "shear" compromise of the nerve. Since this is a chronic process, the nerve frequently is deformed. This is a fairly common cause of unilateral sciatic radiculitis in patients with normal plain x-rays and myelograms. © Charles V. Burton, M.D.

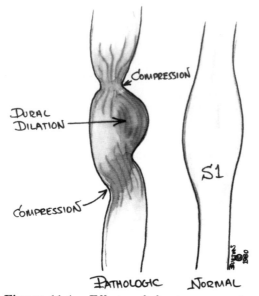

COMPRESSION

DURAL DILATION

S1

COMPRESSION

PATHOLOGIC   NORMAL

Figure 11.4. Effects of facet compression: This drawing is of a case of left S1 nerve root and ganglia compression due to a "superior articular process syndrome." At surgery, the deformations reflected the edges of the superior articular process. Between the areas of insult, the dura was dilated and appeared as a "blue dome cyst." The areas of pressure were markedly erythematous and the dura was laced with tortuous dilated venous varicosities. © Charles V. Burton, M.D.

advent of quality high-resolution CT performed and interpreted by qualified professionals, it has now become possible to accurately diagnose and treat this very important health care problem. It has now become evident in the author's practice that high-resolution CT is not only optimal for the diagnosis of stenosis, but has also replaced myelography as the diagnostic procedure of choice for other pathologic processes.

Nerve compression from lateral spinal stenosis usually produces more pain and less neurologic deficit than prominent disc herniations. While the nature of the process producing pain is not exactly understood, it appears to involve the following factors: (1) interruption of axoplasmic flow, (2) interruption of neurohumoral transport mechanisms, (3) stimulation of fine sensory nerve

endings by distended membranes, (4) anoxia from decreased arterial supply, and (5) engorgement due to impaired venous return.

Although the pathologic nature of lateral spinal stenosis was predicted by a small group of pioneering physicians over the past 28 years, it is only now, due to advanced CT imaging technology, that patients can be objectively evaluated for this entity and have this information translated into appropriate surgical resolution.

LUMBOSACRAL ADHESIVE ARACHNOIDITIS (LSAA)

Arachnoiditis represents a nonspecific inflammatory response by one of the most sensitive tissues of the body. The existence of this pathologic entity has only recently come to the attention of the surgeon. The entity is deserving of careful study and reflection on the basis of the information that LSAA is the primary organic pathology in 6–16% of all FBSS patients[5] and is probably present to some degree in most of all other cases. It is also an entity which usually can be avoided by the physician.

On the basis of many years of study, it is the author's firm belief that while many foreign bodies have the potential to produce LSAA, it is iophendylate (Pantopaque®) which has been the primary etiologic factor in its production in our patients over the past 50 years.

Although the pathology of LSAA has been well documented, the nature of its causation, to some extent, remains unclear. At this time, what *is* clear is that the process involves a number of factors, of which the following appear to be essential: (1) a primary inflammatory focus, (2) foreign body, (3) blood in the cerebrospinal fluid, and (4) autoimmune response.

Figures 11.5–11.8 show in diagrammatic form the basic process. The normal relationships of nerve root, dura, and associated leptomeninges are shown in Figure 11.5. In Figure 11.6, a compressive lesion (i.e., disc)

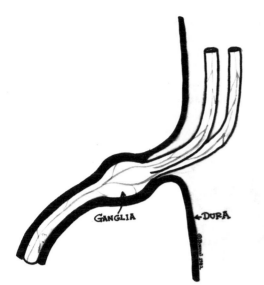

Figure 11.5. Nerve rootlet relationships: A schematic representation of the motor and sensory nerve rootlets fusing to form the dorsal root ganglia is shown. © Charles V. Burton, M.D.

has produced nerve swelling and has initiated an inflammatory response characterized by early fibroblast proliferation and collagen deposition. If the compressive focus is removed, a return to a near-normal resting state will occur. In Figure 11.7, the combination of blood and foreign body maintains and enhances the inflammatory response—even if the original focus is removed. Nerve swelling and hyperemia progress and collagen begins to bind nerve roots to each other and to the lepto and pachy-meninges. It is at this point that the autoimmune effect, alluded to by Mayfield,[7] seems to have greatest significance. Cases in which LSAA have progressed up the neuraxis to involve brain and basilar cisterns have been well-documented.[8]

The final phase characterized by progressive nerve atrophy and the presence of surrounding and intraneural dense collagenous scar tissue is shown in Figure 11.8. At this stage, the dorsal root ganglion is hypersensitive and minimal stimulation produces trains of electrical discharges lasting for many minutes after the initial stimulus.

Scanning electron microscopy of the pia-

arachnoid after exposure to iophendylate consistently shows permanent tissue injury and inflammatory response. Recent tissue culture studies on arachnoidal cells[9] further document the high level of iophendylate toxicity.

There are clearly many agents which may constitute a foreign body to the pia-arachnoid. It seems that the remittent presence of free blood is capable of producing LSAA. There is a little known pathologic entity which was originally described by Foix and Alajouanine[10] as "ascending subacute phlebitis of the spinal cord" which probably represents bleeding into the subarachnoid space from venous abnormalities producing arachnoidal reaction.

Intrathecal steroids have been used for many years to treat lumbar pain as well as a number of neurologic disorders, of which multiple sclerosis is an example. Of particular interest has been the intrathecal injection of methylprednisolone acetate, prepared as a suspension (Depo-Medrol®), as

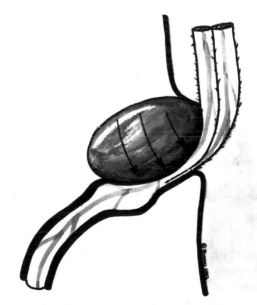

Figure 11.6. Poststenotic swelling: A compressive lesion has produced pre- and poststenotic nerve and ganglion swelling. Impairment of venous return has caused engorgement. Slight fibroblastic proliferation along the nerves has been initiated. © Charles V. Burton, M.D.

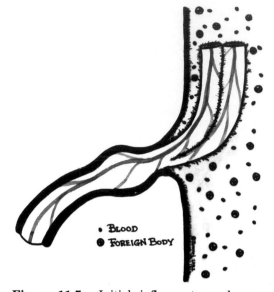

Figure 11.7. Initial inflammatory changes: Although the inflammatory focus has been removed, the inflammatory reaction has been maintained and amplified by free blood in the cerebrospinal fluid, the presence of a foreign body, and the initiation of an autoimmune reaction. Fibroblast deposition of collagen has progressed to the point where the nerves now are adherent to each other. © Charles V. Burton, M.D.

a means of decreasing the meningeal inflammation reaction produced by iophendylate; particularly since Depo-Medrol® itself is etiologic in the production of arachnoiditis. Depo-Medrol® represents a suspension of the steroid in a solution of polyethylene glycol (a nonionic detergent) and myristyl-gamma picolinium chloride (a long-chain fatty acid). There is now substantial evidence that the primary foreign body reaction is not due to the steroid but to the adjuvants.[11, 12]

It is evident that the subarachnoid space is particularly sensitive to irritants and foreign bodies. Even the intrathecal injection of nonpreservative-containing sterile water or isotonic saline produces a brisk cerebrospinal fluid pleocytosis. There is clearly a spectrum of reactivity and many of the water-soluble contrast agents have shown a propensity in this regard with lowest risk

belonging to some of the newer contrast agents such as metrizamide. From the standpoint of highest risk (by many orders of magnitude) and greatest clinical injury over the longest period of time, iophendylate is clearly in a class by itself.

With safer, and more accurate, lumbar myelographic and noninvasive imaging techniques now available, there simply is no legitimate reason to expose a patient to iophendylate. Its demise is now in progress but cannot occur quickly enough. This author is certain that its disappearance will be matched by the absence of iatrogenically induced LSAA.

In summary, it can be stated that while any foreign body has the potential to produce arachnoiditis, there now remains no doubt that it is iophendylate which has been the primary reason for the existence

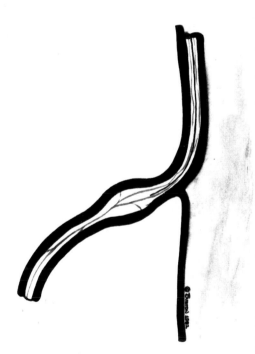

Figure 11.8. Subsequent fibrotic changes: The acute inflammatory phase has subsided and the final phase of the arachnoidal reaction has been reached. The nerves are now atrophic and enmeshed in solid collagenous scar tissue. They are densely adherent to each other and to the meninges. © Charles V. Burton, M.D.

of clinically significant LSAA in the United States.

When adhesive arachnoiditis is considered to be a primary reason for the FBSS, there presently exists little possibility that direct surgical intervention will produce long-term benefit. The author's experience with the intradural removal of scar tissue by tedious microsurgical dissection employing collagen digesting enzymes has not been encouraging enough to recommend it. A number of destructive procedures have been employed (cordotomy, rhizotomy, and ganglionectomy) in the search for pain relief, but there is also little evidence to suggest that long-term relief occurs and there is much evidence to suggest that nerve destruction ultimately leads to pain enhancement through the deafferentation process.

It is in cases of LSAA that the use of implanted electronic pain relief devices seems to be most effective; this procedure is useful in selected patients undergoing comprehensive pain treatment programs conducted by knowledgeable and trained physicians in institutions with appropriate facilities. In recent years, the percutaneous epidural neurostimulating system has become the standard initial means of testing for pain relief in arachnoiditis patients at our Institute. When a good result is obtained on a trial basis, the system may be permanently internalized or replaced by a more definitive dorsal cord neurostimulator. Patient surveys[13, 14] conducted since 1972 by the author consistently have shown a 45–55% good to excellent result in properly evaluated patients.

EPIDURAL FIBROSIS

After surgery, it is the local accumulation of blood in proximity to dura and nerves which promotes fibroblast proliferation and allows the formation of epidural scar tissue. Is this tissue friend or foe? Clearly fibrosis is necessary to promote union of wounds and is the means by which the overlying muscles are rejoined. Epidural fibrosis also is capable of producing fixation of neural elements and, in some cases, actual compression.

In 6–8% of FBSS cases, epidural fibrosis represents the primary organic pathology.[5] Because of high-resolution CT, the nature and extent of epidural fibrosis can be objectively documented. The scan shown in Figure 11.9 is typical for a postlaminectomy study. The extensive epidural scar tissue shown is obviously not beneficial to the patient. Although scar can be removed by microdissection, it is difficult to justify reoperation based on a diagnostic study alone. Those cases which have been operated upon by the author, as part of a comprehensive rehabilitation effort, have shown well-defined sciatic radiculitis and have shown reasonable postsurgical improvement when careful microsurgical dissection and autogeneous full-thickness fat grafts were also employed.

HERNIATED NUCLEUS PULPOSUS

When accurate and complete diagnostic testing reveals a herniated intervertebral lumbar disc as the only significant cause of spinal nerve compression, William of Occam's principle of parsimony is applicable. Basically, this 14th century Franciscan monk stated that, "it is needless to do with more when less will suffice." Surgery should represent the last consideration after the trial of effective, more conservative therapy. With gravity lumbar traction (described later) and chemonucleolysis now available, the physician's armamentarium has been expanded considerably in this regard. One cannot be a FBSS statistic if one has successfully avoided surgery. When surgery is clearly indicated for the treatment of a herniated disc, a situation which probably applies to about 5% of patients presently undergoing surgery, it must be based on accurate and *complete* information. Myelography alone is incapable of providing adequate information regarding the

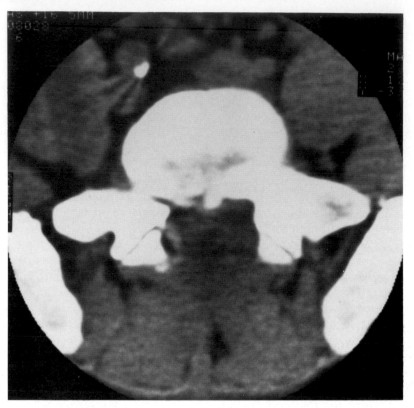

Figure 11.9. Epidural fibrosis: A postlaminectomy high-resolution CT scan shows dense and extensive dorsal and ventral epidural fibrosis.

possibility of coexisting pathology beyond the central canal. The value of high-resolution CT with capability of soft-tissue differentiation is well illustrated by the following case:

J.W., a 52-year-old ex-construction specialist experienced incapacitating back and left leg pain over a 13-year period. He was found to have a prominent left sciatic radiculitis on examination. Previous diagnostic workups at other institutions had failed to reveal the etiology of the problem, and the metrizamide myelogram at our Institute also was normal (Fig. 11.10). High-resolution lumbar CT scan clearly demonstrated a laterally situated disc herniation within the intervertebral foramen (Fig. 11.11). A left L4–5 lateral partial facetectomy allowed removal of a chronic freely protruded disc with

reactive fibrosis, which had produced marked compression of the exiting L4 nerve root. After surgery, the patient has been pain-free for 2 years of follow-up.

CENTRAL SPINAL STENOSIS

The absence of a normal volume spinal canal is a clear liability for the individual in whom disc protrusion or lateral spinal stenosis is in progress. Canal size can be documented by ultrasound and has a valuable predictive value regarding risk for future low back problems.

FUSION OVERGROWTH

Fusion overgrowth is now recognized as a reason for FBSS. It can produce both central and lateral spinal stenosis. While partial fusion take-down for nerve de-

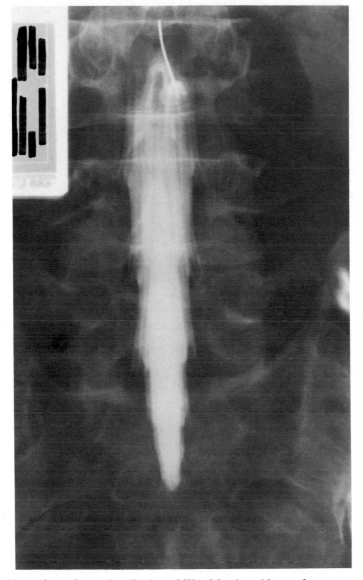

Figure 11.10. Normal myelography (Patient J.W.): Metrizamide myelogram study was considered to be within normal limits.

compression is an arduous task, demanding skill and care to avoid damaging nerve tissue, it is now a routine procedure at our Institute. A more commonly seen complication of fusion is a "transitional syndrome" occurring at the segment above the fusion where accentuated stress has enhanced degenerative disease of the facet joints, producing a localized mechanical low back pain syndrome.

CONSERVATIVE MANAGEMENT

The key to an adequate conservative management program is an accurate diagnosis and application of specific treatment modalities based on this diagnosis. While there are general principles applicable to all patients (weight reduction, low back education, appropriate exercises, psychologic and medical-social support, etc.), specific

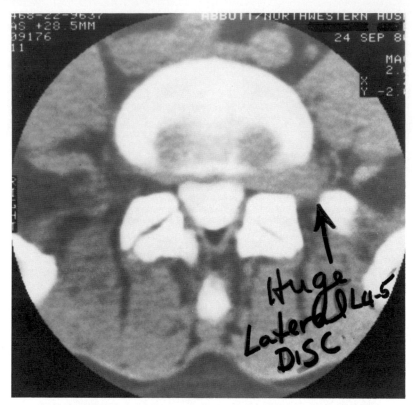

Figure 11.11. Abnormal CT scan (Patient J.W.): High-resolution CT scan shows "huge" laterally protruded disc at L4–5. A free fragment of disc with chronic reactive tissue was found and removed at surgery. The exiting L4 nerve was markedly deformed. The study has been "enhanced" with metrizamide. The facet joints show degenerative disease. There is no indication of lateral spinal stenosis.

early treatment is available, allowing the patient to return to normal function as soon as possible. This approach avoids the liability of disuse atrophy of body tissue, anxiety, frustration, and the sociolegal aspects of workers' compensation sagas. To initiate therapy, an initial attempt is made to determine if the problem is musculoligamentous or primarily related to involvement of a posterior or anterior spinal nerve root.

POSTERIOR NERVE ROOT SYNDROME

Involvement of sinuvertebral or articular posterior (sensory) nerve roots produces characteristic patterns, marked by poorly defined, deep aching pain in the lumbar area, buttocks, or posterior legs. Symptoms related to articular nerve irritation at the zygoapophyseal joints may be alleviated by spine mobilization and temporary facet joint nerve blocks. These patients often may be permanently relieved of pain by multilevel bilateral permanent radiofrequency nerve blocks, the effect of which is to decrease sensitivity of the facet joints, but not to eliminate cutaneous sensation.

ANTERIOR NERVE ROOT SYNDROME

The herniated intervertebral disc producing neurologic deficit is the classic example of the anterior nerve root syndrome and the symptoms are familiar enough to obviate the need for further description. When only the annulus fibrosus and posterior longitudinal ligament are deformed, the symptoms are consistent with a posterior nerve root syndrome. Since less than 5% of anterior nerve root syndromes are surgical emergencies, the average patient is a candidate for conservative treatment. The problem with the usual recommendation of 2–3 months of bed rest is that this approach is impractical and unaffordable by most members of today's dynamic society. Accordingly, the staff of the Sister Kenny Institute has developed a shorter and more practical means of unloading the spine and allowing reduction of the disc and providing nerve decompression. It has been termed the "Gravity Lumbar Reduction Therapy Program" (GLRTP)† and has shown efficacy in about 70% of selected, previously unoperated patients having an *acute contained disc herniation*.[15] In this program, which is accompanied by patient education and physical reactivation, the patient is fitted with a chest harness and is progressively tilted, over an 8- to 10-day period, in a self-controlled electrical tilt bed (Fig. 11.12). After this, the patients are discharged to return to normal activities and to continue either 60° or 90° traction for 1 hour twice a day for 6–12 months (Fig. 11.13).

While GLRPT can serve as the definitive mode of therapy, it has also shown considerable value in demonstrating, in a short period of time, those patients who are surgical candidates. These patients usually have freely extruded disc fragments or fibrotic discs in which gravity traction only increases the pre-existing nerve compression. GLRPT is an example of a new generation of innovative conservative treatment programs presently available to the medical profession.

There is presently a renewed interest in the enzyme chymopapain as an effective means of treatment in selected patients. While not innocuous, chymopapain has

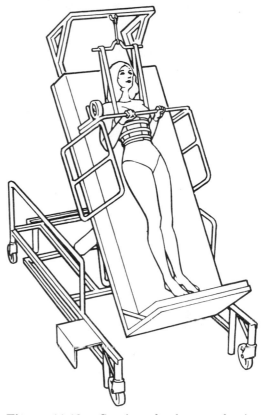

Figure 11.12. Gravity lumbar reduction therapy (acute phase): The patient controls this electrically operated bed. The vest fixates the rib cage which is used to support body weight. Over an 8-day period, the patient advances the angle of traction 5% per day. Each episode of traction is usually 30 minutes. Total time in traction each day is about 4 hours. Note: Safety strap not shown. Reproduced with permission of Sister Kenny Institute.

shown significant promise as a valid therapeutic modality. Safety and efficacy are still under study in the United States under "double-blinded" research protocols which should help determine chymopapain's limitations and true liabilities.

SUMMARY

Through the study of FBSS patients, it has been possible to identify recurring situations in which errors in diagnosis and treatment have been made in the past. The

† GLRTP information is available from Camp International, Jackson, MI.

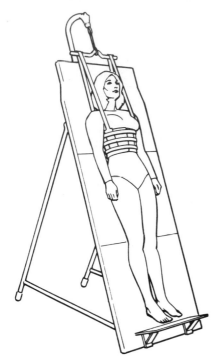

Figure 11.13. Gravity lumbar reduction therapy (post-hospitalization phase): After discharge from the hospital, the traction is maintained for 1 hour twice a day for 3–6 months. Patient returns to normal activities during this treatment phase. Units can be set from 45° to 90°. In the illustration, the patient is using traction at 60°. Note: Safety strap not shown. Reproduced with permission of Sister Kenny Institute.

present availability of more objective, safer, and noninvasive diagnostic tests has allowed complete and accurate initial patient evaluations. This new approach is unquestionably a boon to the low back patient and may serve as the avenue to a more enlightened therapy in the future.

References

1. Gempel, P. A.: Arthur D. Little Decision Resources, quoted in: *Orthopaedics Today 1:*2,4, 1981.
2. Tobias, A.: *The Invisible Bankers.* The Linden Press. Simon and Schuster, New York, 1982.
3. Antonakes, J. A.: Claims cost of back pain. *Best's Review* (Property/Casualty Insurance Edition) *82:*36–129, 1981.
4. Bunney, B. E., Pert, C. B., Klee, W., Costa, E., Pert, A., Davis, G. C.: Basic and clinical studies of endorphins. *Ann. Intern. Med. 91:*239–250, 1979.
5. Burton, C. V., Kirkaldy-Willis, W. H., Young-Hing, K., Heithoff, K. B.: Causes of failure on the lumbar spine. *Clin. Orthop. 157:*191–199, 1981.
6. Verbiest, H.: A radicular syndrome from developmental narrowing of the lumbar vertebral canal. *J. Bone Joint Surg. 36-B:*230–237, 1954.
7. Mayfield, F. H.: Spondylosis and the low back. *Clin. Neurosurg. 37:*345, 1979.
8. Burton, C. V.: Lumbosacral arachnoiditis. *Spine 3:*24–30, 1978.
9. Mayfield, F.: Personal Communication, 1982.
10. Foix and Alajouanine: La Myelite Necrotiquie Subaigue. 1926. Cited in: Diseases of the spine and spinal cord. In: *Greenfield's Neuropathology.* Year Book Medical Publishers, Inc., Chicago, p. 680, 1976.
11. Dellcrud, K., Moreland, T. J.: Adhesive arachnoiditis after lumbar radiculography with Dimer-X and Depo-Medrol. *Radiology 119:*153–155, 1976.
12. Bernat, J. L., Sadowski, C. H., Vincent, F. M., Nordgren, R. E., Margolis, G.: Sclerosing spinal pachymeningitis: A complication of intrathecal administration of Depro-Medrol for multiple sclerosis. *J. Neurol. Neurosurg. Psych. 39:*1124–1128, 1976.
13. Burton, C. V.: Dorsal column stimulation. *Surg. Neurol. 4:*171–175, 1975.
14. Burton, C. W.: Implanted devices for electronic augmentation of nervous system function. *J. Med. Instrumen. 9:*221–223, 1975.
15. Burton, C. V., Nida, G.: The Sister Kenny Institute Gravity Lumbar Reduction Therapy Program, Sister Kenny Institute Publication No. 731, 1976.

Suggested Readings

I. LUMBAR CT SCANNING
1. International Society for the Study of the Lumbar Spine, Symposium: Computed tomography of the lumbar spine. *Spine 4:*282–378, 1979.
2. Post, M. J. D.: Radiographic evaluation of the spine: Current advances with emphasis on computed tomography. Masson Publishing USA, Inc., New York, 1980.
3. Heithoff, K. B.: High-resolution computed tomography of the lumbar spine. *Postgrad. Med. 70:*193–213, 1981.

II. LATERAL SPINAL STENOSIS
1. Kirkaldy-Willis, W. H., McIvor, G. W. D.: Spinal stenosis. *Clin. Orthop. 115:*2–144, 1976.
2. Kirkaldy-Willis, W. H., Wedge, J. H., Yong-Hing, K., Reilly, J.: Pathology and pathogenesis of lumbar spondylosis and stenosis. *Spine 3:*319–328, 1978.
3 Ciric, I., Mikhael, M. A., Tarkington, J. A., Vick, N. A.: The lateral recess syndrome: A variant of spinal stenosis. *J. Neurosurg. 53:*433–445, 1980.
4. Keim, H. A., Kirkaldy-Willis, W. H.: Low back pain. Clinical Symposia. Vol. 32, No. 6, published by Ciba Pharmaceutical Co., Summit, NJ, 1980.

III. FUSION OVERGROWTH

1. Kestler, O. C.: Overgrowth (hypertrophy) of lumbosacral grafts causing a complete block. *Bull. Hosp. Jt. Dis. 27:* 51–57, 1966.
2. Brodsky, A. E.: Postlaminectomy and postfusion stenosis of the lumbar spine. *Clin. Orthop. 115:* 130–139, 1976.

IV. LUMBO-SACRAL ADHESIVE ARACHNOIDITIS

1. Burton, C. V., Wiltse, L. L.: Editorial and symposium on lumbar arachnoiditis: Nomenclature, etiology and pathology. *Spine 3:* 23–92, 1978.

V. EPIDURAL FIBROSIS

1. Benoist, M., Ficat, C., Baraf, P., Caudroix, J.: Postoperative lumbar epiduro-arachnoiditis: Diagnostic and therapeutic aspects. *Spine 5:* 432–436, 1980.

VI. CONSERVATIVE MANAGEMENT

1. Kelsey, J. L., White, A. A.: Epidemiology and impact of low back pain. *Spine 5:* 133–142, 1980.
2. Burton, C. V.: Developments in the treatment of low back pain. *Audio-Digest Orthop.* Vol. 3, No. 4, April 1980. Audio-Digest Foundation (California Medical Association, Glendale CA, 1577 E. Chevy Chase Drive, Glendale, CA 91206).
3. Finneson, B. E.: *Low Back Pain.* 2nd Edition. J. B. Lippincott Co., New York, 1980.
4. Burton, C. V.: Conservative management of low back pain. *Postgrad. Med. 70:* 168–183, 1981.

VII. THE FAILED BACK SURGERY SYNDROME

1. Crock, H. V.: Observations on the management of failed spinal operations. *J. Bone Joint Surg. 58-B:* 193–199, 1976.

VIII. HEALTH CARE ECONOMICS

1. Burton, C. V.: Computed tomographic scanning and the lumbar spine. Part I: economic and historic review. *Spine 4:* 353–355, 1979.
2. Burton, C. V.: Neuroradiology and computerized tomographic scanning. In: *Hospital Special Care Facilities.* H. Laufman, (Ed). Academic Press, New York, 1981.

12

How to Avoid the "Failed Back Surgery Syndrome"*

In 1975, a neurosurgical survey[1] indicated that about 117,000 lumbar operations were performed in the United States each year. When orthopaedic statistics are added, it would be reasonable to estimate a yearly total of 400,000 such procedures in this country. From a review of the past literature on operative success, Nachemson[2] has indicated an overall improvement of only 70% by the first procedure, 30% by the second, and 5% by the third. When one considers the large numbers of surgical failures and the resultant incapacitation and economic burden existing for these unfortunates and for society in general, a persuasive argument for reassessment and improvement of surgical efficacy in this area becomes apparent.

From the viewpoint of a neurosurgeon who has been intimately involved in the diagnosis and "salvage" rehabilitation of thousands of failed back surgery syndrome (FBSS) patients, the author has been in a unique position to discover errors and to recommend changes. The low efficacy of lumbar spine surgery has been studied over a 10-year period and some of the conclusions reached should be meaningful in returning a higher degree of both early and late success to this common operative procedure.

It has been the author's remarkable and consistent observation that lumbar spine surgery has been held in relative contempt as being "easy" and unworthy of serious care and consideration by many surgeons who basically earn their professional livelihood from this endeavor. In fact, skillful back surgery requires the highest level of the physician's diagnostic acumen and technical expertise. Disregard has probably reflected ignorance. Now, with new knowledge and understanding, it is evident that we are emerging from a "dark age" of diagnosis and treatment. A primary problem has been the lack of appreciation of the *actual* living anatomy of the lumbar spine. Through the advent of high-resolution computed tomography (CT), anatomic details can be determined accurately on a case-by-case basis. It has been this lack of reliable and comprehensive preoperative information, as well as the lack of an accurate and noninvasive means of *monitoring* the anatomic result of surgery which has been responsible, in the greatest degree, for past therapeutic failure. Without an accurate diagnosis, no therapy is capable of achieving a reasonable level of success.

There was a time in neurosurgery when brain tumor diagnosis was based completely on the neurologic examination. During that period, some frontal lobe lesions could not (on this basis alone) be differentiated from those in the cerebellum. In many ways, today's diagnosis of low back pain by neurologic examination alone is comparable in its inability to provide a *neurologically specific* diagnosis. CT has

* The author would like to express his deep appreciation to A. Earl Walker, M.D. for the opportunity of learning neurosurgery and to Drs. Frank Otenasek, John Chambers, Neal Aronson, and Richard Otenasek for the practical knowledge inherent to successful surgery and patient care.

proven to be an invaluable aid in clarifying those details in the history and physical examination which are pertinent to the patient's problem. Treatment is never based on a diagnostic study alone. The surgeon's overdependence on myelographic defects has marked a period which has not been medicine's finest hour.

Far too frequently, an FBSS patient's history documents a short period of improvement followed by the return of ipsilateral or contralateral symptoms. Through an experience of about 10,000 high-resolution lumbar CT scans at our institution, the author and his associates have become aware of the bilateral presentation of lumbar degenerative disc disease. A recent study by Chu[3] has shown that 61% of patients with unilateral radicular symptoms evidenced *bilateral* radicular involvement on EMG electrodiagnostic studies. Frequently, the clinical symptoms reflect only the most advanced aspect of a bilateral or multisegmental disease process. The decision to perform spine surgery also should involve this awareness.

It can no longer be considered acceptable for a qualified and experienced surgeon to operate on the lumbar spine unless the following considerations are satisfied:

(1) The diagnosis must be accurate and provide effective treatment for the immediate problem.

(2) Iatrogenic disease is avoided during surgery (this is in particular reference to lumbosacral adhesive arachnoiditis and excessive epidural fibrosis).

(3) At the time of surgery, *impending* problems must be identified and addressed from a prophylactic standpoint.

CLINICAL HISTORY

This remains the single most valuable means of determining the general area in which the patient's problem lies. From history alone, back pain due to extraspinal disease often can be detected. History provides important clues to differentiate musculoligamentous from mechanical syndromes, and these from syndromes involving irritation/compression of mixed spinal nerves. By completing a comprehensive questionnaire including a pain drawing, the patient can provide the physician with valuable information at the initial interview.

PHYSICAL AND NEUROLOGIC EXAMINATION

High-resolution CT with soft-tissue differentiation capability has provided the author with a greater appreciation of what to look for in the physical and neurologic examination. The presence of tenderness of the sciatic nerve at the sciatic notch and in the popliteal fossa in a reliable patient has become an observation of importance, along with motor deficit, "crossed" positive straight leg raising, reflex change, and sensory abnormality. Of inestimable value is the experienced examiner's judgment as to the degree of organic versus functional disease and the ability to "double-check" all abnormalities.

DIAGNOSTIC STUDIES

It now seems unlikely that patients will come to surgery in the future without the benefit of quality high-resolution CT having soft-tissue differentiation capabilities. CT has already made epidural venography obsolete and has replaced myelography as the diagnostic procedure of choice in the lumbar spine.

Water-soluble myelography continues to be the contrast study of choice, both as a primary study and also for CT enhancement. The known potential dangers of iophendylate (Pantopaque®) in patients with lumbar disease is such that it should not be used except in the most unique circumstances.

Newer imaging technology utilizing nuclear magnetic resonance, positron emitted transverse tomography, and advanced display systems will clearly enhance future diagnostic acumen.

SURGICAL TECHNIQUE

Each lumbar operative procedure should represent a unique endeavor based on the presenting pathology and a detailed anatomic study of the patient's spine. Adequate exposure, minimal tissue injury, a dry operative field created by careful hemostasis, magnification, and high-intensity illumination are keys to clinical success. These considerations appear to create low wound infection rates. At our institution, a wound infection rate of less than 1% was reduced to essentially nil by the adoption of the single dose preoperative use of intramuscular tobramycin and intravenous vancomycin advocated by Malis.[4]

Patient positioning to avoid abdominal compression is the single most important preoperative measure leading to a dry operative field and controlled lumbar spine surgery. The modified Tarlov position[5] shown in Figure 12.1 avoids compression of abdominal viscera and the creation of "sway back" seen with other "free abdomen" positions. The liberal use of bone wax has avoided problems from potential air embolism. This is something which must always be guarded against, although the

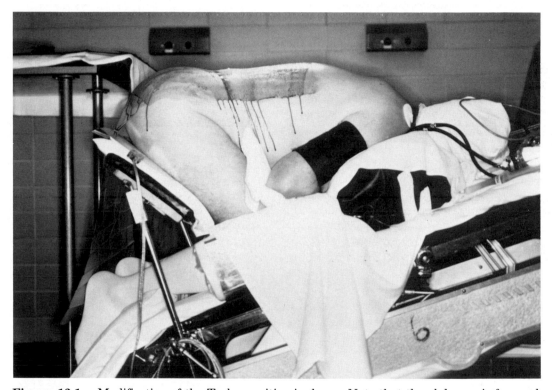

Figure 12.1. Modification of the Tarlov position is shown. Note that the abdomen is free and lumbar spine is not hyperlordotic (sway back). Head elevation can produce pooling of blood in the lower extremities. Thigh-high compressive stockings are used to help avoid this. Knee flexion must not be excessive and peripheral blood flow in the feet must be checked. Wide adhesive tape should be placed across the soles of the feet and attached to the operating room table. Arms are folded under the abdomen (as shown) or placed at the patient's side. Foam rubber pads are utilized to protect all areas of contact (seat, under and lateral to knees, and around arms). Arm extension beyond the head has been abandoned as it caused transient brachial plexus palsies in a few patients. The foam block under the chest must not compress the neck as a transient Horner's syndrome has been noted under this circumstance.

author has never experienced this problem with the Tarlov position.

Magnification and high-intensity illumination are essential requirements for the spinal surgeon. In Figure 12.2, 4.5X operating telescopes with an 18-inch focal point are being utilized with a fiberoptic headlight. This magnification allows the differentiation of dural edge from posterior longitudinal ligament and the use of microsurgical technique to separate epidural scar tissue from nerve tissue. The simplicity and facility of this combination has served the author well for over a decade. Resort to an operating room microscope has been a rare event although microsurgical technique and instrumentation are employed routinely.

"Microsurgical discectomy" can be ade-quately performed utilizing the aids shown in Figure 12.2. It is the author's opinion that while this approach may be valid in young patients in whom the only pathology is a single level, free fragment disc herniation, this is a procedure which is frequently misused. The ideal candidate for microsurgical discectomy represents the atypical disc problem. Application of this procedure in patients with narrow spinal canals or facet entrapment syndrome has been criticized as inadequate treatment.[6]

Manual instruments have a significant advantage over powered tools. They allow the surgeon important "biofeedback" from the senses of hearing and touch. This is particularly true of small osteotomes which have been utilized more often by the author. Osteotomes, rongeurs, curettes, and

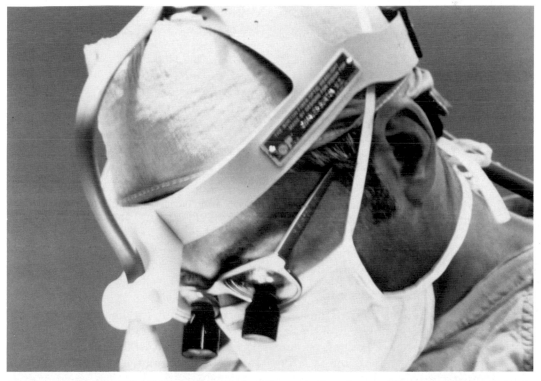

Figure 12.2.   Magnification and illumination: The operating glasses utilize the Galilean telescopic principle (Designs for Vision, New York City, NY) in order to allow higher magnification and greater depth of field-in-focus than loupes. They are mounted so that the surgeon can choose between normal vision with ambient light and magnification. The telescopes shown are wide field 4.5X. Magnification from 2.5X to 9.0X is available, and the point of magnification focus is usually aligned with the fiberoptic beam.

microsurgical instruments occupy the positions of primary use. The author prefers the air turbine drill,† utilizing larger burrs at lower revolutions per minute in order to avoid "chatter" which represents a loss of control and the potential for nerve injury. The air drill is utilized to remove bone mass in proximity to a nerve but hand or sonic curettes are always utilized to remove bone immediately in contact with nerve tissue (Fig. 12.3).

From this author's perspective, the greatest problem encountered by the inexperienced or inadequately trained spinal surgeon is uncontrolled epidural hemorrhage. While proper positioning is essential to reduce abdominal and epidural intravenous pressure, the ability to effectively use cottonoid patties and bipolar coagulation will allow a dry operative field. The result is controlled and effective surgery. Quite frankly, there has been little attention paid to the control of hemorrhage in the past, reflected by operative reports indicating blood losses of 1000–5000 cc. With the technical aids described, it would be unusual for a multilevel "re-do" laminectomy to involve a blood loss of more than 300 cc. Low blood loss allows for rapid and more effective surgery, early patient ambulation, and significantly less morbidity.

The author's present surgical technique has been developed over many years and presently bears little or no resemblance to that which was advocated during his training as a neurosurgical resident at Johns Hopkins University School of Medicine in the 1960's.

With the exception of those few cases where a microsurgical or limited unilateral exposure is justified on the basis of limited pathology, the majority of patients coming to this surgeon's attention require a *bilateral* approach to adequately address the disease process.

This is due to two factors: the rapid advance of more conservative modalities, of

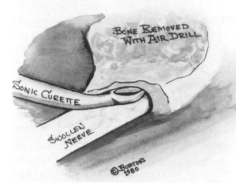

Figure 12.3. Removal of compressive bone: The low speed air drill has removed the main mass of compressive bone. A manual or sonic curette is then used to remove the thin shelf of bone in direct contact with nerve tissue. © Charles V. Burton, M.D.

which the Sister Kenny Institute Gravity Lumbar Reduction Therapy Program and chymopapain for chemonucleolysis are prime examples, and the increasing awareness of degenerative disc disease as a *bilateral* process. Patients presenting with strictly unilateral symptoms are often shown by high-resolution CT to have *impending* contralateral disease.

Figure 12.4 illustrates the basic single level bilateral approach to a lumbar segment. This exposure allows nerve decompression within the spinal canal as well as the lateral recesses. The basic surgical rule of starting from both normal anatomy and a reliable point of reference is essential. Figure 12.5 depicts the author's basic "zipper" approach (bilateral superior hemilaminotomy), where a small osteotome is used to remove the superior edge of a lamina to gain access to the dorsal dura and also to "turn-up" the ligamentum flavum. This approach is quick and safe and is of particular value in establishing normal dura as a reference point in a procedure on a previously operated patient when most of the reference points have been obscured by dense collagenous scar tissue. The segmental exposure is completed by the "horseshoe" maneuver (Fig. 12.6) in which an air drill is used to define the leading edge of

† Information regarding the Minos air drill is available from the 3M Corporation, Minneapolis, MN.

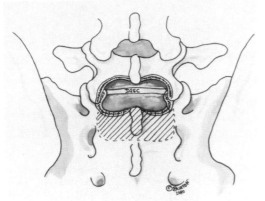

Figure 12.4. Operative approach: Basic single-level exposure for a bilateral approach. This constitutes a bilateral inferior hemilaminotomy and medial facetectomy. The latter may be emphasized on the side of dominant pathology, depending on the anatomy of the zygapophyseal joints. In cases involving S1 nerve roots, the *cross-hatched area* may be removed for more adequate exploration and decompression. © Charles V. Burton, M.D.

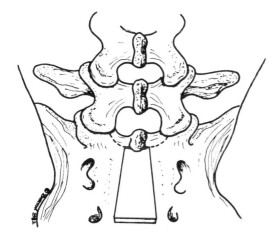

Figure 12.5. The "zipper" approach removing the superior aspect of the dorsal process and bilateral lamina. A narrow manual osteotome is repeatedly driven into bone along the *dotted line*, gradually increasing penetration. As the instrument nears the canal, a definite hollow sound is heard. The "zipper" serves as an effective means of entry to the canal and, as the bone fragment is turned superiorly, the attached ligamentum flavum also is reflected away from the canal. © Charles V. Burton, M.D.

the medial aspect of the inferior articular processes and lamina of the superior vertebrae (bilateral inferior hemilaminotomy). A horseshoe-shaped segment of bone is turned down by repeated use of an osteotome and then a curette. When the zipper and horseshoe are combined, the ligamentum flavum can be removed in toto. An associate of the author, Charles Ray, prefers the use of an electric reciprocating saw to an osteotome and, in some cases, replaces the removed bone segments after decompression. A similar approach has been

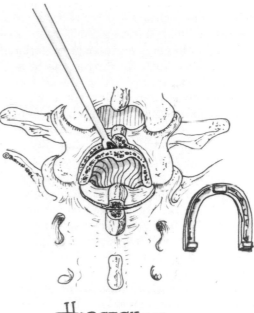

Horseshoe

Figure 12.6. The "horseshoe" maneuver has been performed and the curette is turning down the segment of bone with attached ligamentum flavum. When bone and liagmentum are removed, the medial aspect of the superior articular process of the inferior vertebrae is exposed, and then is resected carefully under direct vision. Care must be taken to maintain the structural integrity of the pars interarticularis. The resulting exposure allows undercutting of the lamina and the superior articular process to the degree necessary to perform nerve decompression. Most helpful in this regard are 6–8 mm wide curved osteotomes and curettes. © Charles V. Burton, M.D.

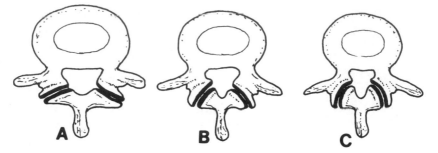

Figure 12.7. So-called normal and symmetrical joints are L5-S1 (A), L4–5 (B), and L3–4 (C) levels. In actuality, the joints are often asymmetric, abnormally oriented, and degenerative. The surgeon *must* appreciate the joint geography so that the operative approach will reflect this information so as to maintain segmental stability.

described by Keim[7] as preparation for bilateral intertransverse process fusion procedures.

The technique described can be initiated at any spinal level. Starting at the S1 segment allows one to identify the S1 nerve root, which is characteristically more medial and dorsal than L5. Another advantage is the opportunity to perform a medial facetectomy when the facet joint anatomy allows this without *creating instability*. A basic principle of the author's surgical technique is to provide nerve decompression *without promoting additional segmental instability*. In this way, decompression without the need for fusion is accomplished.

In order to decompress and avoid instability, the surgeon must study (from CT images) the detailed anatomy of the zygapophyseal joints. Figure 12.7 shows the normal joints at the last three lumbar levels. Many patients with lumbar degenerative disc disease have asymmetric and hypertrophic facets. In *A*, medial facetectomy can be safely performed. In *C*, medial facetectomy would enhance instability; fusion in conjunction with decompression would have to be considered. As can be seen from Figure 12.8, it is also possible to decompress exiting spinal nerves by enlarging the intervertebral foramen (also allowed by the basic exposure).

It is particularly important in treating lateral spinal stenosis that the foramen be enlarged and that patency be documented

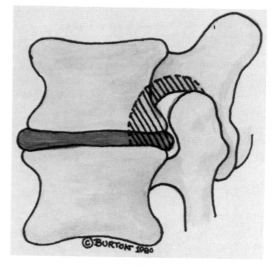

Figure 12.8. The *cross-lined* zone indicates the areas of bone and disc which can be removed by the surgeon to enlarge a compromised intervertebral foramen and not add to segmental instability. © Charles V. Burton, M.D.

by surgical probes or appropriate catheters (Fig. 12.9). The adequacy of nerve decompression can be determined postoperatively by a CT assessment of the foramina, if appropriate.

Once the surgeon has achieved adequate decompression of neural elements and has acted prophylactically to protect the patient from impending pathology, additional concerns must also be addressed. One of the most important of these is the avoidance of severe epidural fibrosis. From the previous chapter, it can be appreciated that

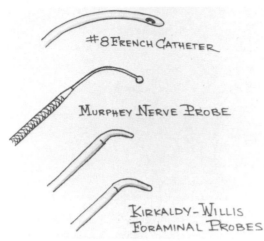

Figure 12.9. Foraminal probes: Commonly utilized probes and catheters used to determine foraminal patency. A #8 plastic pediatric feeding tube with internal stylet has been found quite useful. The Murphey nerve probe is also of significant value as a blunt dissector. The Kirkaldy-Willis foraminal probes have the advantage of graduated size, thus allowing a direct measurement of the foraminal opening.

epidural fibrosis can be a primary etiology for the FBSS. Fibrosis is required for normal wound healing, but its dense adherence to dura and nerve roots is clearly undesirable.

The modern search for a means of preventing epidural fibrosis seems to have been initiated by Lexer[8] in 1919. Many investigators have explored the use of various autologous tissues as well as silastic polymers, gelatin film and foam, microfibrillar collagen, and micropore tape.

Due in large part to the investigations of Mayfield,[9] Kirkaldy-Willis, Yong-Hing et al.,[10] Keller et al.,[11] Gill et al.,[12] Jacobs et al.,[13] and Langenskiold and Kiviluoto,[14] it has become evident that autologous fat was the substance of choice to avoid epidural fibrosis, but a great deal of confusion existed regarding the nature of the graft and preferred means of application. In 1977, the author and his associate, Charles Ray, initiated a fat graft study in which follow-up was carried out by high-resolution CT scans. In one group of patients, particulate fat was taken from the incisional site and placed over exposed nerve roots and dura. After 2 years, high-resolution CT scans showed no significant difference from ungrafted patients in regard to the presence

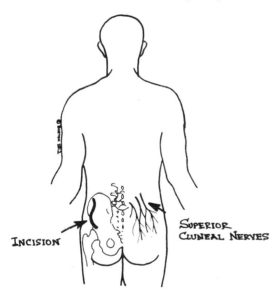

Figure 12.10. Removal of full-thickness fat graft: A "lazy S" incision (to dissipate lines of postsurgical contracture) is made below the crest of the ilium and lateral to the cluneal nerve complex. After graft removal and after careful hemostasis, the skin may be sutured directly to the gluteal fascia to avoid a postoperative "dead space." © Charles V. Burton, M.D.

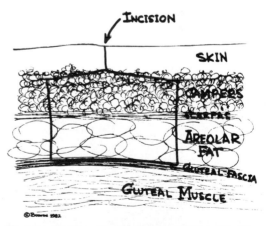

Figure 12.11. Configuration of fat graft: The en-bloc fat graft includes Camper's fascia and the loose areolar fat layer. About 20–30 cc of fat is removed for a major multilevel exploration and decompression. © Charles V. Burton, M.D.

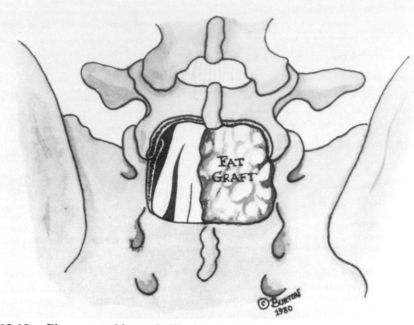

Figure 12.12. Placement of fat graft: The loose areolar fat usually is placed over the nerve roots (and occasionally under them if they are totally exposed after decompression) and the remainder of the graft (the Camper's and Scarpa's layers) are then placed over the dura and loose areolar fat as shown. © Charles V. Burton, M.D.

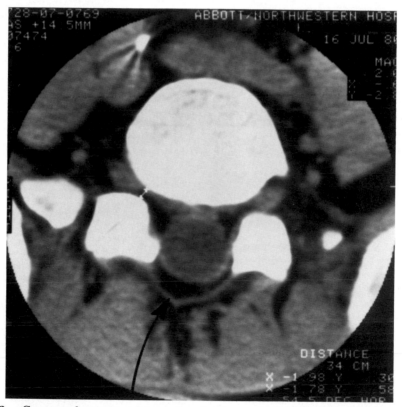

Figure 12.13. Computed tomographic study: A 28-month CT follow-up is shown. Minimal epidural fibrosis is present anterior to the nerve roots and dura. The fat graft is intact and a pseudoligamentum flavum has formed (*arrow*).

of extensive epidural fibrosis. The second group, which consisted of 183 patients, underwent fat grafting from a separate incisional site (Fig. 12.10). The en-bloc graft (Fig. 12.11) is usually 20–30 cc in volume and was placed directly over exposed nerve elements (Fig. 12.12).

By the end of 1981, 32 patients had undergone a 2-year follow-up CT scan to analyze the status of the fat graft and five patients required surgical re-exploration, at which time the fat grafts were inspected and biopsied. In the full-thickness graft series, the findings were essentially the same in all cases. The grafts were intact and had substantially reduced epidural fibrosis. Figure 12.13 shows a representative follow-up scan and Figure 12.14 summarizes the observations. The biopsy specimens were histologically similar to normal fat.

This study has confirmed the impression that fat is the postsurgical material of choice for prevention of undesired epidural fibrosis and that a full-thickness graft taken from a separate incisional site is superior to thinner sections taken from the margins of the laminectomy incision.

CONCLUSIONS

The experience gained by salvaging FBSS patients has provided new insights which can lead to safer and more effective lumbar surgery. One means of documentation has been a review of the surgical success in patients in which a specific and definable organic entity (usually lateral spinal stenosis) was identified and addressed. The author does not wish to imply that these patients were "cured" or did not require additional rehabilitative measures but, as showed in Table 12.1, the clinical success was about 10–15 times better than that previously reported. There is every reason to believe that if these surgical prin-

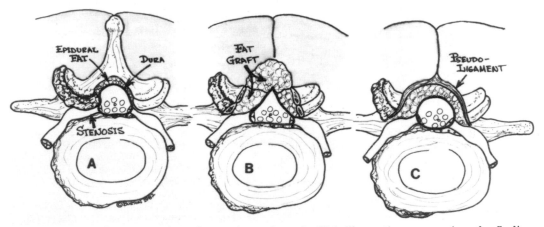

Figure 12.14. Summary of autologous fat graft study: This illustration summarizes the findings of the study. In A, the normal anatomy on the *right* is compared to a case of lateral spinal stenosis on the *left*. In B, decompressive surgery has been carried out. Note the undercutting of the superior articular process on the *left*, allowing the nerve and ganglia to be freed of compression. Loose areolar fat overlies the nerve roots and compresses the dural sac. The major portion of the graft overlies grafts and dura. At the time of wound closure, there is no residual dead space to allow for the accumulation of blood. After 2 years, the volume of grafted fat has decreased about 40%. The dura has re-expanded and a pseudoligamentum flavum has formed between the graft and the paraspinal muscles. The fat is vascularized and histologically similar to normal fat. (Caution: When re-exploring a patient with a full-thickness fat graft, there is a definite danger of dissecting periosteal elevators "slipping" because of the lubricating qualities of the graft. Approach with extra care.) © Charles V. Burton, M.D.

Table 12.1. Clinical efficacy survey 1977–1981: all major lumbar surgery cases

FAILED BACK SURGERY SYNDROME

(225 cases)

Of these patients, the average number of surgeries before being seen was 1.96 per patient. About 80% of these cases were workers' compensation and 31% of these patients had previous fusions.

Objective data available on 194 cases (86%)

160 (83%) improved
27 (14%) unchanged
7 (3%) worse

Subjective data on 201 cases (89%)

147 (73%) improved
22 (11%) unchanged
32 (16%) worse

Drug use on 201 cases (89%)

160 (80%) decreased use
18 (9%) unchanged
23 (11%) increased use

Activity level on 201 cases (89%)

130 (65%) increased activity
33 (16%) unchanged
38 (19%) decreased activity

ciples are applied routinely by lumbar surgeons, the incidence of FBSS should be reduced dramatically and the basic success rate for lumbar spine surgery substantially increased.

There is little doubt but that the *need* for lumbar surgery can be substantially reduced by public low back educational programs, preventive low back care, risk identification programs, and early, aggressive, and effective conservative treatment programs.

SUMMARY

When surgery is based on adequate and reliable pathological and clinical information, the patient has the best chance for a good therapeutic result. Surgery must be planned not only to alleviate the immediate problem effectively, but it must also provide measures to prevent impending future nerve compression. Lumbosacral adhesive arachnoiditis and epidural fibrosis now have been identified as significant adverse influences which substantially can be avoided by discontinuing the use of iophendylate as a lumbar myelographic media and routinely employing full-thickness autologous fat grafts from a separate incisional site.

Although high quality, high-resolution CT scans of the spine having soft-tissue differentiation capabilities are not yet routinely available, this imaging modality clearly is destined to become the presurgical diagnostic study of choice (as it is at this time at our Institute). The anatomical, physiologic, and pathologic nature of the human lumbar spine is a subject which is so complex and which has been so little understood in the past, that this individual stands in awe of what he has learned in only the past few years. The author sincerely hopes that his surgical colleagues will share this experience and begin to hold this surgical challenge in the high regard that it truly deserves.

References

1. Neurosurgical Manpower Commission Report: *AANS-MINDS* 72:2308, 1975.
2. Nachemson, A.: Presented as discussion at the International Society for the Study of the Lumbar Spine, May, 1980.
3. Chu, J.: Lumbosacral radicular symptoms: Importance of bilateral electrodiagnostic studies. Presented at the American Congress of Physical Medicine and Rehabilitation, San Diego, CA, December, 1981.
4. Malis, L. I.: Prevention of neurosurgical infection by intraoperative antibiotics. *Neurosurgery* 5:339–343, 1976.
5. Tarlov, I.: The knee-chest position for lower spinal operations. *J. Bone Joint Surg.* 49-A:6,1193–1194, 1967.
6. Davis, C. II.: Personal Communication, 1982.
7. Keim, H. A.: Indications for spine fusions and techniques. *Clin. Neurosurg.* 25:184–192, 1978.
8. Lexer, E.: Die freian transplantationen Part 1. *Neue Deutsche Cirurgie 26*, Stuttgart, Ferdinand Enke, pp. 264–545, 1919.

9. Mayfield, F. H.: Autologous fat transplants for the protection and repair of the spinal dura. *Clin. Neurosurg. 27:*349–361, 1980.
10. Yong-Hing, K., Reilly, J., deKorompay, V., Kirkaldy-Willis, W. H.: Prevention of nerve root adhesions after laminectomy. *Spine 5:*59–64, 1980.
11. Keller, J. T., Dunsker, S. B., McWhorter, J. M., Ongkiko, C. M., Saunders, M. D., Mayfield, F. H.: The fate of autogenous grafts to the spinal dura. *J. Neurosurg. 49:*412–418, 1978.
12. Gill, G. G., Sakovich, L., Thompson, E.: Pedicle fat grafts for the prevention of scar formation after laminectomy. *Spine 4:*176–186, 1978.
13. Jacobs, R. R., McClain, B. S., Neff, J.: Control of postlaminectomy scar formation: An experimental and clinical study. *Spine 5:*223–229, 1980.
14. Langenskiold, A., Kiviluoto, O.: Prevention of epidural scar formation after operations on the lumbar spine by means of free fat transplants. *Clin. Orthop. 115:*92–95, 1976.

Index